PRAISE FOR *TAKING CHARGE OF*

"Lupus is such a misunderstood disease. It's great to see a comprehensive book for understanding and living with lupus. This book is new and different in its approach to helping everyone understand lupus and the effects it has on friends and family members. Maureen Pratt and David Hallegua have created an informative, compassionate read for patients and families dealing with the challenge of lupus."

> —Mary McDonough, Actress and President of Lupus LA

"I have many, many friends with lupus. I know firsthand that it can be a baffling and challenging disease to live with. *Taking Charge of Lupus* is an important book—interesting, clear, informative. Maureen Pratt and Dr. Hallegua have taken the mystery out of lupus, which will help a patient cope better and lead a healthier and more productive life."

> —Carrie Brillstein, President of the Executive Committee, Lupus LA

"This book is a remarkable journey for a doctor and a patient. Simply stated, Pratt and Hallegua demonstrate that a knowledgeable and informed patient together with a compassionate and experienced physician can make a difference. Lupus is not a death sentence, and the self-efficacy displayed by the advice given in this book will actually improve the outcome for the patient. The information contained in this volume will be of enormous help to our patients."

> —Michael Weisman, M.D., Chief of Rheumatology,
> Cedars-Sinai Medical Center in Los Angeles, and
> Professor of Medicine, UCLA School of Medicine

TAKING CHARGE of LUPUS

TAKING CHARGE of LUPUS

How to Manage the Disease and Make the Most of Your Life

Maureen Pratt and David Hallegua, M.D.
Foreword by Daniel J. Wallace, M.D.

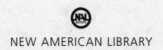

NEW AMERICAN LIBRARY

New American Library
Published by New American Library, a division of
Penguin Group (USA) Inc., 375 Hudson Street,
New York, New York 10014, U.S.A.
Penguin Books Ltd, 80 Strand,
London WC2R 0RL, England
Penguin Books Australia Ltd, 250 Camberwell Road,
Camberwell, Victoria 3124, Australia
Penguin Books Canada Ltd, 10 Alcorn Avenue,
Toronto, Ontario, Canada M4V 3B2
Penguin Books (N.Z.) Ltd, Cnr Rosedale and Airborne Roads,
Albany, Auckland 1310, New Zealand

Penguin Books Ltd, Registered Offices:
80 Strand, London WC2R 0RL, England

First published by New American Library, a division of Penguin Group (USA) Inc.

First Printing, September 2002
10 9 8 7 6 5 4 3 2

 REGISTERED TRADEMARK—MARCA REGISTRADA

LIBRARY OF CONGRESS CATALOGING IN PUBLICATION DATA:

Pratt, Maureen.
Taking charge of lupus : how to manage the disease and make the most of your life /
Maureen Pratt and David Hallegua ; foreword by Daniel J. Wallace.
p. cm.
Includes index.
ISBN 0-451-20699-1 (alk. paper)
1. Systemic lupus erythematosus—Popular works. I. Hallegua, David. II. Title.
RC924.5.L85 P735 2002
362.1'9677—dc21   2002069230

Set in Janson
Designed by Ginger Legato

Printed in the United States of America

PUBLISHER'S NOTE
Every effort has been made to ensure that the information contained in this book is complete and accurate. However, neither the publisher nor the authors are engaged in render-
ing professional advice or services to the individual reader. The ideas, procedures, and suggestions contained in this book are not intended as a substitute for consulting with your
physician. All matters regarding your health require medical supervision. Neither the
authors nor the publisher shall be liable for any loss or damage allegedly arising from any
information or suggestion in this book.

While the authors have made every effort to provide accurate telephone numbers and
Internet addresses at the time of publication, neither the publisher nor the authors assume
any responsibility for errors, or for changes that occur after publication.

Contents

Foreword

Taking Charge of Lupus, a protean effort by a gifted patient, Maureen Pratt, and a Renaissance physician, David Hallegua, merits your attention. It distills years of experience into an easy-to-read and understandable road map for both recently diagnosed lupus patients and longtime lupus sufferers. The authors do not deal with how lupus is diagnosed or the road to being told one has lupus. Now that you have it, their collective wisdom crystallizes many of the conundrums that confound patients: How does one approach his or her doctor, family, work, relationships, and life in general? Since the head bone is connected to the lupus bone, and one's stamina and endurance are stretched to the limit, how can the lupus sufferer maximize his or her efforts and summon the courage to slay the wolf at his or her door?

Taking Charge of Lupus reminds me of the great medieval philosopher/physician Maimonides' *The Guide of the Perplexed* in that it offers the lupus patient a new, improved form of chicken soup, one of Maimonides' major contributions to medicine. Maimonides also embraced an active approach to illness. In this book, the patient is encouraged to take a proactive stance, for example taking advantage of medical opportunities such as clinical trials, and use the diagnosis as occasion for introspection and self-improvement in order to ultimately come out a better, positive, more spiritual being.

I highly recommend *Taking Charge of Lupus* to all with the disorder.

Daniel J. Wallace, M.D.
Los Angeles, 2002

Acknowledgments

Writing this book has been a wonderful journey, and there are many who, along the way, have helped make it happen.

First, I'd like to thank God for giving me this opportunity to share what I have learned and for His ever-present comfort and strength. I'd also like to thank Dr. Hallegua for his terrific contribution and dedication to this work, and Dr. Wallace for his support and encouragement. My deep appreciation to Father Frank Desiderio, Rabbi Levi Meier, Lisa Waldman, and Carolyn Dodge for their insights on coping, faith, and feelings.

Portions of the chapter on people who care for loved ones with lupus first appeared in articles that I wrote for "LupusLine," a publication of Lupus International, and I'd like to thank Christina Kelly and her staff for their help with them. Also, many thanks to my fellow members of LupusLA for persevering in raising lupus awareness and research funding despite much personal hardship.

To my sisters and brothers in the choir, and Linda, Barbara, Alan, Brian, Ann, Irv, Nancy, Judy, David, Judy, Paul, Jean, Jay, Pam, Nicki, Mary, Libby, Misti, Tim, Carlos, Janet, Amy, Fredi, Jeff, Father Walsh, Marvin, and Elia—all of whom helped shape this book and make it physically possible for me to write it—thank you for *everything*.

To Marie Timell and the team at NAL—you're the best! To Jane Jordan Browne and everyone at MPDInc., well, I can't say enough about how wonderful you've been (and continue to be).

And to my mother, to whom I dedicate this book, I give my biggest of thanks and hugs!

Maureen Pratt
Los Angeles, 2002

At the outset I want to thank Maureen Pratt for including me in this important endeavor and to wish her success in her future efforts and good health and happiness always. I also want to thank all the people who have helped me reach this point in my career but it would take a separate book to include all the many teachers, friends, colleagues, and family members who have shaped my character and enriched my knowledge during my life.

What I can do is thank the people who were instrumental in helping me with this project, such as Dr. Wallace, who supported the writing of this book and whose work has never ceased to inspire me. I am also grateful to my wife, Cici, for enduring the late hours while I was writing this book and for her helpful validation and editing.

David S. Hallegua, M.D.
Los Angeles, 2002

INTRODUCTION

You Have the Diagnosis. Now What?

You have lupus.

The waiting and the wondering are over. Your doctor has finally confirmed your diagnosis: Your pain and strange symptoms are not products of your imagination. Rather, you have a definite disease.

Upon receiving the news, you probably feel a mixture of emotions. First among them may be shock and fear that you have an incurable illness. But you may also feel a profound sense of relief that your symptoms are finally recognized as something other than psychosomatic or mystifying. And you are not alone in having that reaction. Because lupus wears so many different guises, and because the ability to diagnose it requires specific and perceptive application of clinical observation and other signs and symptoms, lupus often goes undiagnosed. It is not unusual for a patient to suffer from multiple symptoms for several years before her or his medical team figures out that all those roads point to lupus. You might know this firsthand; perhaps your own road to diagnosis was long, frustrating, and physically painful. However, the good news is that now you know. You have lupus. And that's a better place to start than where you were before the diagnosis.

Along with being relieved, you may believe that, now that you know what is wrong, you can begin to treat your disease, or even cure it. That is natural—we live in an era when medical breakthroughs and miracles occur every day. The solution for many ailments seems so easy: Go to your doctor. Take a pill. Use an ointment. Take a month off work. You'll be cured.

It must be the same for lupus, right?

Or you might hear stories from friends, acquaintances, even anonymous e-mails, assuring you that this or that new treatment will cure you once and for all. Many of these treatments are expensive, some more harmful than helpful. But if the end result is a cure, they must be worth it, right?

Unfortunately, as of this writing there is no cure for lupus. But there are new treatments and diagnostic procedures that are more refined and sometimes less invasive than those used in years past. There are ways to make life more livable with lupus, too; that is, there are tangible things that you and your loved ones can do to ease the stress, pain, and frustration that come with a chronic illness. With advance planning, you can also take away some of the sting of the inevitable surprises that lupus will bring into your life.

What Does Lupus Mean to Me?

After the relief of putting a definite name to your disease, and the comfort of knowing there may be some treatment for your symptoms, you are, no doubt, full of questions.

- What exactly is lupus?
- Will you have to give up parts of your life? How will your disease affect work? Sports? Travel? Dreams? Goals?
- What do you say to others, who understand your disease even less than you do?
- How can you ensure that your health care is the best it possibly can be?
- How do you enter into relationships with your health-care providers that are supportive and encouraging, not stifling?
- How will living with a chronic illness affect your relationships with loved ones and coworkers?

Yes, amid the turmoil, there is good news: Although lupus is a difficult disease to live with, and there is no cure yet, you need not live in despair. Your fellow "lupies" (and their loved ones) find fulfillment and even joy in their lives each day, in spite of their disease. You can, too!

1

Some Facts about Lupus

What Is Lupus?

Although it is not rare, lupus is not a widely known disease. Here are some basic facts: Lupus is an autoimmune disease in which the body becomes "allergic" to itself, meaning the immune system turns away from protecting the body from infection and cancers and instead begins to attack the body's own tissues and organs.

There are three types of lupus: cutaneous or discoid lupus (DLE), systemic lupus erythematosus (SLE), and drug-induced lupus erythematosus. In DLE, the manifestation of lupus is external (skin, hair, etc.). In SLE, the manifestation can be external and internal. In SLE, any organ can become involved in the autoimmune process. In drug-induced lupus, the disease develops from use of a prescription drug and usually disappears after the drug is discontinued.

Recent Lupus Foundation of America market research data show that up to 2.5 million women, men, and children in the United States share your disease. However, each case of lupus is unique, and each patient suffers from a different combination of symptoms and disease prognoses. Likewise, the treatments used vary from patient to patient, depending on the experience and determination of the treating physician, the patient's symptoms, and the level of drug availability and the patient's tolerance.

Lupus is an autoimmune rheumatic disease. A rheumatic disease is a disorder that affects the immune or musculoskeletal systems.

The physicians who specialize in treating lupus are usually rheumatologists. The American College of Rheumatology (ACR) lists eleven symptoms or signs (criteria) that help facilitate the diagnosis of SLE. The list of criteria does not cover all lupus-related symptoms. However, it does serve as a guide for physicians and other medical professionals who are trying to determine the cause of diverse, often perplexing symptoms. To be diagnosed with SLE, a patient should have four or more of these symptoms; however, the symptoms do not have to occur at the same time (and seldom do). For that reason, lupus patients often go several years before a doctor puts all the pieces of the lupus puzzle together and arrives at a diagnosis of SLE.

Lupus from a Rheumatologist's Perspective

Systemic lupus erythematosus, commonly known as lupus, is the prototype of an autoimmune disease in which the body's defense against infection and tumors mediated by the white cells in the blood turns against and attempts to destroy various organs in the body. Since there is no single symptom, sign, or test that can reliably identify every single lupus patient, the physician must rely on the presence of a combination of symptoms, signs, and tests called *criteria* to establish the diagnosis. Since these signs and tests are found months or years apart, it often takes years and visits to many doctors before a diagnosis of lupus is established.

The majority of the approximately 2.5 million lupus patients in the United States are women in their reproductive years. However, men or people older than sixty-five are not immune to this disease, and some babies born to some mothers with lupus may have transient lupus at birth. About 50 percent of lupus patients have joint pain and 20 percent have skin rashes as their initial symptom. In the rest, the disease may manifest with mysterious fevers, fluid around the heart and lungs, or abdominal pain. A few unfortunate lupus patients have catastrophic illnesses such as seizures, coma, or kidney failure as their initial symptom.

As for the course of the disease, lupus will threaten to cause failure of internal organs such as the kidney, blood cells, brain, heart, or liver in about half of affected patients in the first few years of their illness. The remaining half of patients will have to cope with some form, in varying severity, of joint and muscle pains, fatigue, skin rashes, and cognitive and emotional disturbances for most of their lives, since there is no cure for this illness.

Fortunately, as dire as this may sound, effective treatment can control most of the symptoms and signs of lupus. Since many patients with organ-threatening illness have joint pains and rashes as their initial symptoms, an early diagnosis can help doctors to institute treatments that may prevent serious organ involvement later.

Thus, it is important to promote awareness to physicians and patients alike that joint pain and skin rashes may constitute a "lupus attack." It may, in fact, impart a sense of urgency to treating physicians, who might otherwise adopt a more benign "wait and see" attitude toward the patient's relatively innocuous-seeming symptoms. A physician's willingness to make an early diagnosis of lupus is crucial for this disease that can be fatal if not adequately treated.

The following list is from the ACR (1997), and gives the clinical categories for the criteria. They are not listed in order of importance. Besides the explanation given with each criterion, a glossary on page 209 will help you understand the more technical terms.

The Eleven Criteria

Malar Rash   Raised red rash over the cheeks (a "butterfly-shaped pattern with its wings draped over the bridge of the nose onto the upper cheek area" sparing the tip of the nose—not to be confused with rosacea, an infection of the facial skin glands, or seborrheic dermatitis, which is characterized by scaling and redness in the fold between the cheek and the upper lip).

Discoid Rash   Variably shaped patches with loss of pigment and hair follicles and *often leaving scars* (may occur anywhere on the body).

Photosensitivity   Adverse reaction to sunlight, resulting in the development of or increase in any skin rash (can also precipitate other symptoms, such as fever).

Oral Ulcers   Ulcers in the nose or mouth, usually painless (not canker sores, which are typically painful and red with a yellow margin).

Arthritis   Arthritis that causes pain and swelling, but no bone destruction, involving two or more joints, excluding the spine and joints around the breastbone (arthritis in which the bones around the joints do not become destroyed).

Serositis   Pleuritis (inflammation of the sac around the lungs) or pericarditis (inflammation of the sac around the heart).

Renal Disorder   Excessive protein in the urine (greater than 0.5 g/day or 3+ on test sticks) and/or cellular casts (abnormal elements in the urine, derived from red and/or white cells and/or kidney tubule cells).

Neurologic Disorder   Although almost all patients with lupus have some neurologic disease, such as depression or impairment in concentration or memory, only generalized seizures (convulsions) and/or psychosis, which occur in less than 10 percent of patients, are considered criteria for a neurologic disease. This must occur in the absence of drugs or metabolic disturbances that are known to cause such effects.

Hematologic Disorder	Red cell breakdown causing anemia, which is a decrease in the oxygen-delivering red cells in the body. Decrease in the white cell count or leukopenia below 4,000 cells per cubic millimeter of blood or lymphopenia (less than 1,500 lymphocytes per cubic millimeter). These cells protect the body against infection. Thrombocytopenia (less than 100,000 platelets or clotting cells per cubic millimeter). The leukopenia and lymphopenia must be detected in the absence of drugs known to induce it.
Immunologic Disorder	Antibodies normally protect against infections. In lupus, abnormal antibodies develop that are harmful to one's own cells. Examples include a positive LE prep test, and a positive antidouble-stranded DNA antibody that is directed against one's own DNA, or a false positive syphilis (VDRL) *or* phospholipid antibody test, which indicates an increase in the tendency for the blood to clot.
Antinuclear Antibody	Positive test for antinuclear antibodies (ANA), which are antibodies directed against the contents of the nuclei of the cells, in the absence of drugs known to induce the antibodies.

Lupus and You

Lupus patients are, the saying goes, as different as snowflakes. Symptoms may take on many forms, and the course of the disease is different for each patient. So someone with SLE may have a consistently mild course of disease (not to be confused with "not painful" or "not life altering") with no serious organ involvement at all. Someone else may have "silent" lupus, where the effects on internal organs are not felt, but only determined by lab tests. Still another lupus patient might experience a course of disease that "hops" from the skin to the sac around the heart to the gastrointestinal tract and back again!

Truly, this is an unpredictable disease that often can sneak up on a patient. One longtime lupus patient even says it is like "living with a terrorist." Any way it is described, lupus is life changing.

As if the disease were not tricky enough, different patients react differently to the various medicines and procedures used to treat the symptoms. New drugs become available, too, adding more possibly unforeseen reactions into the mix. It might take several tries to find the right combination of medications, or to assemble the medical team that will work best in your situation. Side effects may take years to develop, or may occur immediately.

Again, don't despair. Just be patient. There are many medications available (and different ways of administering the same medications), and new procedures and treatments being developed every year. For example, if one anti-inflammatory doesn't work, there are many others available. If a gym exercise program doesn't bring relief, there is pool exercise.

Be open to alternatives within the purview of your doctor's guidance and recommendations. And stay hopeful. Attitude means a great deal when it comes to overall health.

What about Men with Lupus?

Though only one out of ten patients with lupus is male, the disease usually tends to be organ threatening and debilitating more often than in women. The fatigue and joint and muscle pain that accompany lupus curtail these young men from fitting in with their more active colleagues. Treatment with steroids such as prednisone has the effect of shrinking muscles, the opposite of the affect of anabolic steroids frequently used by bodybuilders.

Since most men with lupus have organ-threatening illnesses such as kidney disease, chemotherapy medicine such as cyclophosphamide is often required. This may lead to premature hair loss, sterility, and impotence, and appropriate steps to store sperm and limit the cumulative dose of chemotherapy must be taken.

Wives of affected lupus patients often have to work to support the family, which can lower the male lupus patient's self-esteem further and cause depression. Children, especially sons, may have a difficult time adjusting to their father's illness and his inability to play outdoor games with them.

What Factors Contribute to the Development of Systemic Lupus?

There are many genes that act together with nongenetic environmental stimuli to determine the person's susceptibility to systemic lupus. Only 50 percent of identical twins are concordant for lupus. In other words, if one twin in an identical twin sib pair has lupus, the chance of the other twin having lupus is only 50 percent, though they share 100 percent of the same genes. This suggests that other factors in the environment play an important role in determining susceptibility.

Complement gene deficiencies such as C1q deficiency (a protein that helps to clear antibody complexes from the circulation) is very rare but gives a 100 percent likelihood of developing lupus; and other complement gene deficiencies such as C2 and C4 gene deficiency increase the chance for SLE but not to 100 percent. Yet other genes and gene deficiencies have been found that predispose patients of different ethnicities to kidney involvement. Isolating the genes from areas of the cell DNA that appear to be similar across lupus patients is an area of active research.

Common environmental agents such as ultraviolet light from sunlight have been conclusively shown to be triggers for lupus in clinical experiments and in practice. Other agents such as hair dyes, infectious pathogens, and drugs may play a role, although the exact significance of these agents is still not clear. Programmed cell death that occurs in the body on a continual basis can function as a stimulus for the immune system to direct antibodies against oneself. Slow clearance of the by-products of cell death in the presence of unregulated immune cell overactivity can sustain immune-mediated damage to the tissues of the body.

2

Taking Control of the Quality of Your Life Despite the Challenges of Lupus

The Road Less Traveled

Beyond the medical aspects of the disease, lupus brings with it significant changes in lifestyle, abilities, dreams, and goals that must be dealt with. Although you might feel helpless at all the changes that might occur in your life, there are some things you can do to reach a certain degree of comfort with the new life you must carve out.

Lupus = Change

Change is an alteration in the regular course of events, the difference between the way things were and the way things evolve. Everyone, whether young or old, lupus patient or not, experiences change throughout life. To live is, in and of itself, to change.

That said, lupus patients must deal with a different kind of change than they had expected before their diagnoses. The disease causes changes that are completely new and sometimes frightening to the patient and his or her loved ones. Things happen to and around the lupus patient that he or she never even imagined.

How a patient copes with change will directly impact his or her health, as well as every other aspect of life. At the onset of your disease, you would do well to take stock of how you approach change, what emotional responses you feel when something is beyond your control, and the degree to which you try to make the most out of a difficult event or situation.

Discerning what to do when life as it was goes awry is a significant challenge, and one that unfolds throughout the rest of life, through all the highs and lows, calm times and flares. This includes redefining your personal quality of life, setting goals in an uncertain world, and moving ahead even if faced with setbacks. Another formidable challenge is finding a new peace of heart and soul, and maintaining it as your body and life continue to go in unexpected—and sometimes frightening and painful—ways.

Changes Specific to Lupus

The greatest and most difficult changes due to lupus are those that affect the body, inside and out. These changes can be abrupt, painful, even life threatening. And they occur at a time when other, "normal" people in the patient's peer group may find it difficult to empathize.

For example, most people believe they will probably someday get arthritis; have to cope with heart, lung, or kidney problems; or lose their hair, hearing, or eyesight. But not at age twenty-two, thirty-five, or even forty-seven. And yet, most lupus patients are diagnosed and first experience their symptoms during their child-bearing years.

Other changes involve the emotional life of a lupus patient, and his or her relationships with loved ones, strangers, and self. The patient can experience mood swings due to fear of the unknown, chronic pain, or medication reactions, and may appear to change overnight. Likewise, those who love people with lupus might find their own ability to cope with difficult times alters as they discover that lupus is chronic, and that flares and symptoms will not be cured all of a sudden.

Before diagnosis, women and men engage in relationships as a normal matter of course, taking comfort in the natural order of them (parent to child, child to parent, husband to wife, friend to friend). But after the diagnosis of lupus, these same men and women may find personal relationships challenging. Marriages may fall apart or become so hostile or unsettling that it is as though the loved one has become a different person altogether.

With a diagnosis of lupus, the future, physical and emotional, is less certain. Before diagnosis, someone might have life all mapped out, with a career track going from entry level to top of the heap. But with lupus in the picture, that map takes on a different look, with unforeseen detours and derailments. The financial and professional picture of life is blurry or, perhaps, lying in shattered pieces on the floor.

Spiritually, many newly diagnosed lupus patients experience upheaval, too. Perhaps you have a strong belief in God, and have felt his goodness and love on one or more occasions. Now that you have been diagnosed with a chronic disease, you might find your faith shaken and your perspective on God taking on a warier, even more doubtful hue. Your relationship with your faith community might become strained as you struggle with your internal spiritual turmoil. You might even come to the point where you don't believe in God anymore at all, especially if you feel your life careening down a path that terrifies you.

A Sense of Control

Having control over some aspects of your life is very important when you suffer from a seemingly out-of-control disease. Lupus patients who recognize that they are not completely at the mercy of the disease tend to cope better than those who give in to despair. Loved ones of lupus patients will have a greater sense of security if the patient can and does take control, even if it is of small things.

"Control?" you ask. "There *is* no control."

At first glance, this is true.

From the outset of your diagnosis, you know that lupus is a chronic disease. This means there is no cure. You will have to adapt your life to accommodate your need to battle symptoms, avoid flares, and undergo treatments and medications that are designed to help, but that might even, in some cases, bring on their own painful symptoms, side effects, and/or flares.

In addition to the reality of lupus, your body seems to start calling the shots, telling you how it feels, what it can and cannot do, and what it will and will not tolerate. Your doctor and other health-care professionals tell you what medications to take, what treatments to seek, and what you should not do.

Your loved ones, too, will want to exercise their control over your condition. Probably acting out of fear and love for you, they will insist you let them take care of you, do things for you, and instruct you as to what they think you should be doing (or not doing) to make yourself feel better.

When you are first diagnosed with lupus, or when you have been living with it for a long time and gone through several flares, you might be tempted to throw up your hands and say, "I give up! There's nothing I can do to control this!"

Positive Steps/Positive Results

There *are* things you can do to gain some control over your life. Although they will not cure your lupus, they will give you a better sense of well-being and lead you on to a tolerable quality of life.

For example, what you eat is completely under your control, as are what you wear, how you set your appearance each day, and how much you choose to exercise. Helping your body achieve a healthful state in terms of the nutrients you feed it or the improvements you make to your body image will go a long way to give you more strength to deal with the negative side of what's going on inside and out.

You can also control some of the things that cause you undue stress.

"Anger tends to grow out of feelings of helplessness," says Lisa Waldman, a licensed psychotherapist and educator who works with lupus patients. "The more positive actions you take in your life—whether it's exercising, if you are able, finding volunteer work, getting involved with other lupus patients in a support group, exploring pain-management options, working part-time—the less angry you are likely to feel."

Certainly, deciding to do something that will give you a sense of being productive, then following through with it, is a good way to take some control over your life, even if you are not working at a regular job. It will enable you to believe in yourself all over again, perhaps allowing you to take even more pride and happiness in your accomplishments *in spite of* lupus than you ever did before.

Taking yourself out of harmful situations, even if it will cause dissension between you and a friend, family member, or colleague, is another way in which you can gain control over your environment and, thus, over the things you allow to impact you and your health.

"I cannot stress enough the importance of ridding yourself of the toxic people in your life," says Rabbi Levi Meier, Jewish chaplain at Cedars-Sinai Medical Center in Los Angeles. "You wouldn't think of eating something poisonous, or taking a slow-drip, intravenous dose of poison. Why allow yourself to be slowly 'poisoned' by someone's toxic nature?"

Another way you can take control of your life is to acquire accurate knowledge and use it appropriately. This means carefully sifting through the daily barrage of people and publications that try to sell you on this or that treatment, alternative, or cure. Although their intentions may be well-meaning, the results of diving into what they offer could be extremely detrimental to you. Do not be pulled this way and that by "the latest in lupus," but make use of the expert guidance given by your doctor, as well as your own powers of reasoning, to steer you through all the news.

Some people refuse to see a doctor after their initial flare subsides and symptoms abate. This false bravado can have very serious consequences for the future, when lupus flares again. Lupus requires regular monitoring for effective treatment, even in times of relative remission. It is up to you to take charge of record keeping and of tracking your disease. You have control over whether you follow through with appointments, tests, and treatments.

Just as you take in food to nourish your body, you also control how you nurture your inner spirit. If you find yourself looking at the world negatively, engage in practices that help you to change your perspective to one that is more uplifting. Use positive visualization (picturing how you'd like things to be instead of dwelling on how they are) or positive affirmations (telling yourself that you respect yourself, accept yourself, and are sure that you are loved by God, family, friends, and yourself). Listen to an inspiring piece of music or read a spiritual text to put you in the right frame of mind. Take a walk, if you are able, and enjoy the natural beauty of the world around you—and know that you are as much a part of it as your lupus is!

What Is Your Ideal Quality of Life?

Defining what makes you happy, what gives your life meaning, joy, and comfort, is the first step toward determining your ideal quality of life. It might seem difficult to do this, but in order to take charge of your disease, it is important for you to set and keep in mind your goals. Ask yourself what kind of quality of life you want, given the realities of lupus. This question needs to be answered by you, individually, in order for you to be able to set future goals, as well as to be content with your here and now. Looking at the basic components of what constitutes quality of life will help you get on your way.

- **Peace of Mind**
The degree to which you are able to feel calm in the midst of pain, changes, and unforeseen roadblocks to plans you have made will greatly influence your quality of life. Peace of mind starts with regular practice of taking quiet time away from noise and activity to further nurture your inner spirit. It comes from accepting your situation, and from being comfortable with yourself even when you are alone.

- **Depth of Personal Relationships**
The people in your life (friends and/or family members) to whom you can turn for support, love, and laughter add greatly to your overall quality of life. Personal relationships that lift you up, rather than drag you down, are essential to you as you struggle with the challenges thrown at you by lupus. Also, your ability to be a good friend, wife, mother, sister, or brother will bring you a greater sense of belonging, meaning, and grace.

- **Physical Comforts**
A simple life, one in which your home, belongings, and activities bring you comfort and stability, is vital to establishing a strong foundation in your life. Living within your means, physically, emotionally, and financially, will support you tremendously in the good and bad times. Taking all the noxious possessions and habits out of your life so that you can focus on being well and enjoying yourself is important, too.

- **Health Concerns**
Fear of lupus could interfere with your ability to seek appropriate medical attention or take the right steps to live healthfully. Learning how to understand and talk reasonably about lupus in your life, and communicate your pain, fears, and symptoms to others, will help take away your fear and give you a strong sense of empowerment. Taking care of all aspects of your medical life, including making sure you get the proper treatments and live a healthful lifestyle, are all part of taking charge of your disease, too.

• **Usefulness to Others and the World**

Even if you are in a lupus flare, it is still important for you to feel that your life has meaning and is of use to the world. Being honest about your health and physical constraints will help you gauge what you can do, as will examining what is your heart's desire. Determination to act positively in your life, to make a difference to those around you, will give you focused energy with which to make your activity count.

Setting Goals to Achieve and Keep Quality of Life

Once you have addressed the above areas, you are ready to establish some goals that will help you achieve your desired quality of life and keep it, in spite of lupus flares and other problems. To set these goals, you will need to examine your priorities; in other words, you need to determine what is important for you, what is less so, and what you can live without.

What Really Sparks You?

Productive goals are things that make you want to get up in the morning and work, even in the face of obstacles. A goal set after you are diagnosed with lupus must be especially energizing to you because of the extra struggle you will endure to see it come to fruition.

When you set your goals and reset priorities, think of what is really interesting to you. What do you want to spend those precious "good" hours doing? What is it that really sparks you, makes you forget, if only for a short while, the pain and anxiety that lupus causes?

Is it gardening? Try night gardening, or growing plants indoors.

Is it sports? Explore different indoor sports that you might be able to participate in. If you can't be that physically active, look into volunteering for a sports-related organization, or even think of working with a local team as, say, a timekeeper.

Whatever you choose to spend your time doing, make sure it is nurturing for you, helpful to others, and doable in terms of your health, financial situation, and family responsibilities. Once you've determined this—go for it! The things you achieve will give you an incredible boost of self-confidence and happiness, and most assuredly contribute greatly to your desired quality of life.

Getting Sidetracked but Moving Ahead

One tool that can be very helpful in showing you how far you have come from the day you are diagnosed onward is a lupus diary. In it, you can write about your struggles and triumphs and candidly articulate your fears and frustrations. By enabling you to look back on your early days of coping with the disease, the diary will show you that you can overcome obstacles, develop patience to weather flares, and learn more about yourself in the process.

In fact, lupus patients are probably some of the most self-aware people in the world, with their perceptions of body changes, spiritual depth, and character. This, ironically, is one of the greatest gifts lupus gives. And it will certainly stand you in very good stead when you face setbacks on the way to achieving your beloved goals.

3

The Keys to Maintaining Quality of Life

Necessities of Life with Lupus

There are seven main factors of life that you need to address and be comfortable with in order to achieve your desired quality of life. These factors address key areas pertaining to your health, emotional well-being, work/play activities, finances, relationships, personal life, and faith.

Each factor dealing with a particular area should be balanced gently with the rest, sometimes taking on a more important role, other times less. Taking charge of and keeping these areas of your life in order will help you manage your health and avoid triggers that can bring on lupus flares. It will also greatly reduce your stress, another important element in coping with lupus.

What Triggers Lupus Flares?

Although there are few definitive causes of lupus, there are several triggers that may play a role in weakening your overall health, bringing on flares and/or exacerbating your symptoms once lupus has developed. These include:

- Prolonged exposure to sunlight
- Air pollutants such as cigarette and cigar smoke, smog, and dust
- Illness and infections
- Extreme stress
- Sleep deprivation
- Inadequate medical monitoring of disease activity
- Radical changes in diet
- Excessive amounts of alfalfa, or products processed using alfalfa (this is the only food that has been definitively linked to triggering lupus flares)

Sometimes lupus will flare even if you stay clear of all of the triggers. But oftentimes flares can be prevented or lessened in severity if your exposure to these triggers is carefully controlled. At first this might seem difficult. Perhaps you live in a sunny climate and have enjoyed spending time outdoors. Or you may be a smoker or live with someone who smokes and have difficulty facing the need for you or your loved one to quit. You may be a young parent, and sleep deprivation is part of your role as mother or father.

Some triggers are difficult to avoid, especially if they are environmental, such as smog or inadvertent exposure to infection if you stand next to someone with a cold in a supermarket checkout line.

Still, the more aware you are of your needs as a lupus patient and of your surroundings, the more you will be able to lessen your contact with things that trigger your lupus. Taking charge of the seven factors addressing key areas of your life will help you do this and give you a more positive, healthful outlook. And you begin with addressing how your emotions influence your approach to living with lupus.

The Emotional Factor

Living with the ups and downs of lupus, a chronic disease, might send your emotions on a roller coaster–like ride. How you cope with your feelings will have a direct impact on how you manage all other aspects of your disease. If you deny your disease or the symptoms of it, for example, you might not seek timely and appropriate medical care. You could become more ill than you would have if you had acknowledged and accepted your health status.

If you allow anger to grip you, you might drive supportive people away from you and exacerbate your anger, stress, and lupus as a result.

Depression occurs in many lupus patients. Sometimes it has emotional roots and sometimes it can be disease-induced. Either way, it is important to recognize the signs of depression and seek medical help when they arise.

Self-awareness is crucial to healthy emotional functioning, as is developing a vocabulary of feelings that go beyond "happy" and "sad" to encompass the many shades of your feelings. By taking charge of your emotional awareness, you will take charge of other factors influenced by lupus. By being positive about what you can do, you will make great strides toward achieving your desired quality of life.

The emotional support you provide yourself with is, in a sense, emotional medicine, and you need to keep it up-to-date and handy, just as you do with any other medication your doctor prescribes.

The Medical Factor

Perhaps you are the kind of person who has never been ill, until affected by lupus. Or you might have been sick, off and on, for years, and now, with a clear diagnosis in hand, you anticipate a change of health that will enable you to sail clearly through the future. Perhaps you always thought that illnesses were signs of weakness and should be ignored, or pushed through. Or now you might think you must be tough and not give in to pain, fatigue, or other lupus symptoms.

Whatever your medical history or attitudes toward health, there is no way to avoid the fact that having lupus means that you now require ongoing medical monitoring and, often, treatment. Historically, you may not be used to paying your doctors frequent visits, having regular lab work performed, or taking medication for extended periods of time—or for life. You might be unable to find a comfortable way to afford the cost of these things. But ignoring the medical realities of lupus can lead to trouble, sometimes terrible trouble. Disregarding the dangers of being out in the sun, for example, can lead to extreme flares, including seizures. "Pushing through" the fatigue characteristic of lupus can lead to collapse. Stopping medication, without the advice of your doctor, can have dangerous consequences. Shirking doctor appointments altogether may allow unseen conditions to worsen and potentially put your life in jeopardy.

The medical aspects of coping with lupus need to be addressed, and the person most involved with the disease is you. You need to understand that lupus is not a weakness but a disease, and there is help for many, if not all, of the symptoms you will experience. Despite time, financial, and personal constraints, you need to be proactive about setting up a medical team you can develop a rapport with and trust. You need to be disciplined about keeping track of your symptoms, reactions to medications, and questions, so that the team can respond effectively. You must educate yourself about your disease and your response to its treatment to develop trust in yourself. Then you will respond appropriately if lupus flares and have a balanced perspective if you are in a "quiet period."

Finding a way to manage the medical aspects of lupus in your life is not an option. It is key to your well-being from now on.

The Financial Factor

Lupus can have a significant effect upon your finances and financial goals. Medical expenses can rise seemingly overnight as you make doctor visits, take expensive medication, and undergo extensive tests and procedures. Even if you have a "mild," non-organ-threatening disease, you will still need to see a doctor regularly and undergo routine rheumatological blood work and possibly other tests as well.

Your productivity can be affected by the disease, resulting in your having to reduce work hours or file for disability. Your health insurance premiums might rise, or because of your lupus diagnosis, your insurer might drop your coverage altogether.

Planning expenses relating to other areas of finances, such as for education, child rearing, retirement, or long-term care of a parent or spouse, can become seemingly impossible in the face of these ongoing expenses. These financial constraints may affect your emotions, create stress, and exacerbate your lupus.

As soon as you have your diagnosis, you should examine your current financial situation and reprioritize your budget to take into account new, lupus-related expenses. Assess your need for adequate health insurance, a just-in-case provision for reducing work hours or going on disability, and a clear rainy-day plan, on top of your known expenses. If you have a mild disease, you might never need to fall back on these contingency plans. But you can take comfort in knowing you are prepared, come what may.

The Productivity Factor

Having lupus may mean that you are unable to perform at your usual level at work, at home, and within your family or social circle for long periods of time. Leisure activities you enjoyed before could be out of the question. For example, if you were an avid golfer, you might have to give up the game because of your photosensitivity. Tennis and other high-impact sports may be off-limits to you.

If in your work you deal with the public, such as in shops, restaurants, or schools, you might have to stop and look for another job because you can't afford to be exposed to environments that breed germs. The immunosuppressive drugs you take to treat your lupus cause you to be more prone to severe infections. Meanwhile, if your disease includes serious organ involvement, you may have to leave the workforce completely. Long-term career planning could seem completely unfeasible in the face of the unpredictable nature of your disease.

If you have a family, you may feel that lupus robs you of your effectiveness and identity as a mother, a father, or a sibling. You may not have the energy to give to others, and your nights might be so filled with pain that any intimacy with your partner becomes impossible. You also might have to cease involvement in special school, family, or community events due to flares. Keeping the house clean and the garden nurtured might become impossible because of joint pain. You may start to become someone you never thought you'd be, someone unreliable, irresponsible, "out of commission."

Feelings of uselessness, coupled with disease-caused pain, can lead to depression and a feeling that your life is spiraling out of control. Lupus itself can induce depression, too. But you need not come to the point where everything seems hopeless. Keep in mind that, no matter how severe your disease, you are a worthwhile person with much to give to yourself and others. Retooling your skills to cope with your illness so that you can feel productive may take time and patience, but is possible. Finding ways to translate that realization into action is key to achieving a level of productivity that can sustain your talents, dreams, and affections through the hard times when lupus takes over.

The Personal Factor

The physical changes caused by lupus and, sometimes, the medications used to treat the disease can deeply affect your self-esteem. Hair loss, weight gain, skin rashes, and decreased energy can contribute to the feeling that you are unattractive, uninteresting, and incapable of being of any benefit to self or others. It is important for you to understand the changes taking place inside and outside your body and take steps to make them more bearable—even enjoyable (yes, wearing wigs can be fun!).

Learning how lupus works and what medications' potential side effects are can help increase your awareness and enable you to take the appropriate medical steps to mitigate them. Being creative with your makeup and clothing can give you a tremendous sense of empowerment and make you more comfortable in the world outside of lupus.

You can control your intake of food, giving your body the best fuel you can. You can also explore new ways to get essential exercise to make sure you retain your range of motion and build stamina.

Having lupus doesn't mean you'll have to give up your dreams of traveling, having children, or succeeding in your profession. You might just have to find more creative ways to accomplish these goals, in spite of and with your lupus.

The Relationship Factor

Of all the resources available to you, perhaps the most obvious are the people with whom you associate. Family, friends, coworkers, acquaintances—all are important to you and have influence over the tone of your life. Yet they might be even more confused than you over what your diagnosis means and how it will affect their relationships with you.

Other people's reactions to your diagnosis might surprise you. Some people will "get it" immediately; they will be willing to adapt to the constraints under which you have to live. They may even offer to help you in your struggle. Others never will. Still others will be partially understanding—sometimes. Unfortunately, you will find that lupus can take a toll on personal relationships.

"This wasn't what I expected when I got married," is a frequent complaint of the spouses of lupus patients. Pressures mount on those married to lupus sufferers. They witness loved ones experiencing hair loss, muscle weakness, weight gain, and the mood swings that go along with a lupus patient on an immunosuppressive drug or prednisone. These pressures tax a marriage, often to the breaking point.

Other relationships suffer, too. Many lupus patients find that their circle of friends diminishes because of the unpredictable nature of the disease. Missing birthdays, weddings, and other celebrations can become too frustrating for some. Coworkers who were once friendly may resent lupus patients because of prolonged absences due to flares and the subsequent heavier workloads they have to take on. Children of lupus patients may have a hard time understanding why Mommy can't participate in school activities, or why Daddy can't coach Little League like the other dads. And parents of lupus patients might fall into complete denial over their child's condition.

Although it is important for a lupus patient to find inner strength, the support and love of others is vital. Just as important is reaching out to loved ones and supporting them, too. Working with family and friends to help them understand lupus and to find new ways for them to cope with how the disease affects you are skills that can be developed, even in the midst of serious flares.

Letting go of people who refuse to understand, or who hinder you from finding peace of mind, is another part of building a fulfilling personal life. Some of this will be done for you; friends will stop calling or issuing invitations because you never seem to be available. But in some cases, you might have to initiate the break, as difficult as it may be. You might have to disengage yourself from a longtime friend who continues to press you to do things that might be harmful for you, such as spending time in the sun. You might need to stop talking with someone who refuses to believe you have lupus, or who believes you did something wrong to bring it on.

With all of this personal upheaval, making new friends, some of whom share your experience with lupus, is one very positive aspect of reaching out and discovering new areas of growth. Another is rediscovering the strength of current relationships, and being able to enjoy them in a new and brilliant light. Lupus can help you see that there is a simple, deep joy in just being with people you care about. And in that, there is much comfort and strength that will help you through the darkest moments.

The Faith Factor

"Have faith."

It's a phrase that is meant to calm a worried mind, and you will probably hear it more than once from people who mean well.

But if you are suffering from lupus, you might find it difficult to embrace this idea, with all of the comfort it is intended to bring. Your physical pain might be too excruciating, your personal disappointment too great to accept this seemingly simple two-word panacea.

"Have faith in what?" you might ask. "In whom? Why?"

There is no cure for lupus, so it is difficult to have faith in the medical community.

When your body is warring against its own tissues, how can you have faith in it? When you can't control your own health, how can you have faith in yourself?

It may also be hard to have faith in God. If you believe that God has a loving role in your life, why would He bring such suffering upon you?

For that matter, why try to have faith at all? Flares will inevitably come and troubles will undoubtedly arise. Won't life with lupus just be one problem after another?

Despite the logic of the above questions, having faith *is* an essential element to coping with lupus. Not to have faith is to be either complacent—which serves no purpose when fighting a disease—or despairing—which is counterproductive to achieving balance and a sense of well-being. Without an active inner life, spiritual focus, belief, and sense of hope, life with lupus can even be dangerous. It can become difficult, if not impossible, to reach out for new treatments, continue relationships with loved ones, and find fresh activities and ways of doing old ones that bring satisfaction.

Without faith, it is impossible to take charge of lupus.

Medical professionals are constantly looking for better ways to treat the symptoms of lupus, and researchers are working at finding a cure. You have innate strength that you didn't know you had, strength that will be revealed and tested by lupus, but needn't be defeated by it. And, rather than severing your communication with a God you feel has let you down, keeping your prayer and meditative life active will help to calm your worries and prepare you for the ups and downs of your newly defined life.

By putting part of your attention and heart into something greater than yourself, you will come to some wonderful insights that are beyond your disease, perhaps even beyond you, thus giving you perspective and the richness an inner life can provide.

Your life with lupus need not be bereft of hope. Rather, the challenges brought on by the disease can deepen your inner life and help you reach a whole new level of awareness of the world around you and your own unique place in it.

Moving Forward

The seven key factors are addressed in more depth in the chapters that follow. In some cases more than one chapter is devoted to a factor. Each chapter offers sound advice and concrete suggestions for taking charge of the specific area of life that a factor addresses. Making so many changes may seem daunting, and you might feel as though you don't have the energy, strength, or fortitude to carry through with them. But if you take your life, and lupus, step by step, you will be able to look back and see you've traveled far and gained much in the way of knowledge, self-awareness, resilience, and peace of mind and spirit.

Life with lupus *is* hard. But it is also full of treasures. And only by moving forward with it will you have the opportunity to discover them.

4

THE EMOTIONAL FACTOR:

How Lupus Affects Your Feelings

In order to take charge of your lupus, you must understand the broad range of emotions that influence your sense of well-being, thoughts, and actions. These emotions are often more acute in lupus patients because of the chronic nature of the disease and the changes, losses, pain, and frustration that accompany it.

Relief, depression, denial, anger, sorrow, hopelessness, and fear are all part of each lupus patient's emotional palette, but so too are joy, triumph, hope, and acceptance. A positive outlook will carry you through your darkest moments and help you make the most of your life, dreams, and goals.

No two cases of lupus are the same. Each lupus patient experiences a different set of symptoms at different times, and the disease progression (or lack thereof) is also unique. Even reactions to medication can vary from patient to patient. There are, however, some similarities and areas of overlap among the experiences of lupus patients, especially in their emotional responses to lupus.

Relief

It might seem odd that a diagnosis of a chronic illness should be met with relief, but that is really one of the first emotional responses the new lupus patient feels. The road to a diagnosis can be long and very painful. There might be years between the onset of the first symptoms and the actual confirmation that there is indeed something medically wrong. Many patients are first told that they are stressed or too busy when they present their physicians with complaints of fatigue, joint pain, and hair loss. Some patients are also told that there is nothing wrong at all, that their discomfort is "all in the head." One lupus patient, whose first symptoms included significant hair loss, was asked by her physician if she might be pulling her hair out herself!

It is no wonder, then, that the lupus patient is relieved when he or she is told that there *is* something medically wrong. A feeling of euphoria might set in as doubt and frustration fall away.

This initial heady sense of triumph that someone has finally listened and confirmed what the patient has known all along might remain for days, even weeks. But do not mistake it for the end of the lupus road. In fact, the journey is just beginning, and the first step in taking charge of it is recognizing that lupus brings loss.

Loss

At the onset of diagnosis and throughout a life with lupus, each patient must cope with a profound and very real sense of loss. This can include loss of health, loss of activities, loss of relationships, loss of financial stability, loss of goals. The phases a patient goes through to cope with these losses are very similar to the stages of grief and include denial, anger, depression, sorrow, fear, and guilt. Because not all of the losses occur or are recognized immediately following diagnosis, the process of experiencing and coping with them is ongoing. Understanding this and practicing vigilance and patience as you work through your reactions will take you a long way toward maintaining a quality of life that is comforting and meaningful.

Denial

As you discover what the reality of a life with lupus means to you, you might slip into denial—denial of the diagnosis, denial of the thought that you will have to make lifestyle changes to accommodate your chronic illness, denial of your own ability to cope. Denial is not a completely detrimental response.

"Denial can be a defense mechanism," says Lisa Waldman. "Denial shields us against unwanted emotions such as anxiety or depression. As a coping mechanism, denial allows you to adjust to the impact of a situation such as lupus, while absorbing the reality in small doses."

Denial can help lessen the shock of hearing you have an incurable, serious illness and, in doing so, relieve you of some of the stress you feel at being diagnosed. However, taken to the extreme, denial can interfere with your ability to cope with your illness and achieve a satisfying quality of life.

Denial might lead you to approach your health-care needs more conservatively. You might decide not to keep doctor appointments, or put off tests necessary to determining the extent of your lupus and the kinds of treatments you must have.

Lupus is a difficult disease to understand, and because there is no definitive lupus test, the criteria for diagnosing it are also seemingly nonspecific. Even with extensive testing and examination, you might deny your diagnosis and think that your doctor has made a mistake, completely refusing to take his or her advice and exacerbating your symptoms as a result. Or you might go from doctor to doctor, hoping you will hear what you want to hear (that you do not really have lupus). Going for a second opinion is prudent and can bring you to the point of deciding to battle your disease effectively. However, going for a third, fourth, or fifth opinion and not really hearing the reality of your condition is not prudent, or healthful, at all.

The Denial of Others

As you tell others of your disease, you will discover that denial is not exclusive to you, the patient. Your loved ones, coworkers, even strangers might doubt that you have lupus, especially if you do not manifest any obvious symptoms of your illness. You will hear comments such as, "I get tired, too. Go to bed a little early and you'll feel better." Or "Won't more aspirin take care of your pain? It helps me when I work out too much." Or "Kidney disease? You're too young."

Most people diagnosed with lupus are women. If you are a man and have been diagnosed, you will undoubtedly hear skeptical comments such as, "I thought only women got lupus," or "You can't have lupus; that's a woman's disease."

If you use a handicap placard for your automobile, someone

might challenge your right to park in a designated handicap space, and you will feel anger, frustration, and confusion about how to respond. Friends might pressure you to "put on a little extra sunblock" and go to the beach with them, despite your telling them that you are sun sensitive. Your children might doubt your illness because of their own fears or because none of their friends' parents are sick all the time. Again, the perception is that if you don't look sick, you can't be sick.

But you know how you feel.

And if the second opinion, your symptoms, and your doctor's assurance point to lupus, the chances are very good that you do have lupus. You cannot control how others react to this fact. You cannot stop others from denying the reality of your condition. But you can control how you react both to others and to your situation. Moreover, you can control what positive actions you take on your own behalf.

The Dangers of Denial

Remaining stuck in denial can have detrimental effects upon your ability to get better physically and take charge of those areas that are within your grasp to control. Ignoring the disease can do more harm than good. There are enough damaging things going on in your body because of lupus; you do not want to bring more trouble upon yourself.

Danger signs of denial include the following:

- Missed doctor appointments
- Stopping medication without a doctor's supervision
- Ignoring symptoms, expecting them to go away on their own
- Prolonging your exposure to the sun
- Partaking in high-impact exercise that puts excessive pressure on sensitive joints
- Consuming inappropriate levels of alcohol
- Smoking
- Refusing to discuss lupus in general and/or the patient's own case
- Testing your limits by retreating from and then returning to previous levels of stressful living

Moving away from Denial: Taking Action

Acknowledging that you have lupus starts with the first talk you have with your doctor upon receiving the diagnosis. Schedule a time when you can meet with your physician and have a specific discussion of your symptoms, test results, course of treatment, and prognosis. Take notes during this discussion (you might even want to tape-record it), and ask questions, even if you think they are minor or stupid.

Keeping your emotions bottled up inside can increase your stress and exacerbate your lupus symptoms. So you must begin to practice sharing your feelings and expressing yourself immediately. This will help bring lupus into your vocabulary and lessen some of your denial, too. The doctor's office is a great place to start.

Gathering information about lupus is also an important step toward acknowledging the presence of the disease in your life. Reading this book and others, investigating Internet sites, and obtaining information from the Arthritis Foundation and the Lupus Foundation of America are all ways to find out more about lupus and connect the disease to your personal experience. A list of helpful organizations is included on pages 211–214.

Keep a log of your symptoms. This will help you keep track of how lupus is affecting you and will help you work with your physician to map out your treatment. Also, in periods when the disease is not active or you fall back into denial, it will remind you that the disease is truly present. This log will come in handy for other reasons, too, which will be discussed later.

If other family members are in denial, ask them to come to a doctor's appointment with you, or make an appointment of their own. Invite them to ask questions and develop their own rapport with the members of your medical team. Understand that it might take them a while to come to terms with your illness, and some of them might never acknowledge it. Throughout this transition period, take care of yourself, even if your loved ones are not on board with your medical condition and treatments.

Once you have been diagnosed, you might want to seek out others who have the disease. Be selective at this stage; you do not want to have horror stories scare you into an inability to start treatment. But having a "lupus buddy" with whom you can talk, share, and learn is a great help.

Support groups can also be excellent sources for information, camaraderie, and validation that you are not alone. Many local chapters of the Arthritis Foundation and Lupus Foundation sponsor support groups for the patient, as well as for "caring others"—loved ones who care for and about lupus patients. Many groups on the Internet host bulletin boards and chat rooms on-line, and these are good cyber–gathering places, especially if you are housebound. A specific discussion of supportive organizations and groups is included in the Appendix at the back of this book.

If you are a caring other and feel that your loved one is denying lupus to his or her detriment, talk to him or her about it. Giving assurance that you care deeply about your loved one's welfare, suggest that he or she reach out to a support group, medical professional, or other trusted individual for guidance. Be firm, constant, and patient. It could take several months or even a few years before the full awareness of a life with lupus sinks in.

The Excellent Lupus Patient

Some personality traits that are common in lupus patients who have prominent autonomic symptoms such as migraine headaches, bowel and bladder disturbances, and Raynaud's phenomenon are the tendency to be an overachiever and to be perfectionistic. Although there is at present no evidence to suggest that having such a personality predisposes one to lupus, it definitely makes it difficult to cope with the vagaries of an unpredictable and chronic illness. The constant striving to achieve mastery and control over one's symptoms and a perfect balance of health leads to a cycle of failure, low self-esteem, and a greater sense of anxiety, anger, and desire to try to achieve perfection again. One is better off trying to achieve excellence rather than perfection, and this can lead to a decrease in anxiety and improve one's self-worth.

Anger

As a lupus patient, it is natural for you to be angry about what has happened to you. This anger may express itself in many ways: rage at the disease, your life, and even the other people in it.

Besides the emotional side of coping with a chronic illness, lupus can often bring physical pain, and that, in turn, can spark angry feelings. Certain medications (corticosteroids in particular) can heighten emotional responses, especially anger. Untangling the web of health insurance reimbursement or obtaining authorization for medical procedures can also bring about frustration, which can lead to anger. Simple daily chores or errands can become aggravating when you add lupus to the mix.

The Dangers of Anger

Although you are certainly justified in being angry with the extra pain and anguish that lupus brings into your life, anger can be harmful. You might become angry at your doctor for not fixing everything, and turn away from essential medical care. You might become angry with God for letting this happen, and break away from your faith at a time when it is most important for you to rely upon it.

Especially if it is acted out in harsh words and physical isolation, anger can put a wedge between you and your loved ones, the very people upon whom you need to rely.

"Anger may be inappropriately displaced onto people in your life, or even strangers, like the local checkout cashier, or onto your doctor—people who don't really deserve it," says Lisa Waldman. "And family members need to be careful not to become angry with the person with lupus for being sick, when they are really angry at the disease itself.

"When anger is not addressed, when it's held in, it can be turned inward and directed against yourself. This is one of the causes of depression," she adds. "Also, efforts to restrict and control anger can cause a buildup of internal stress and frustrations and may, in some people, result in an increase in physical symptoms."

Being angry can drain you of the energy that you need to fight lupus and keep up with your daily activities and responsibilities. You could become unable to take part in daily life because you are so angry, letting your social commitments, work obligations, and everyday chores fall by the wayside. This can create another cycle of stress and, in turn, further exacerbate your lupus symptoms and jeopardize your short- and long-term dreams and goals.

Coping with Anger

Anger management is crucial to coping with lupus. The key is to develop awareness of your feelings, what triggers your anger and when. Carefully examine the reasons for your anger, as well as how you handle it. Recognize and take responsibility for your angry feelings. Try to be as objective as possible, gauging the degree and appropriateness of your reaction to certain situations and emotions. Waldman says, "Review your history of dealing with anger, and that includes exploring family patterns. Also, and this is the hard part, learn to express anger directly and constructively with words."

It is important to express your anger in some way; otherwise it can lead to a debilitating depression. Talking about your anger with people who can handle it can help you get control of this potentially volatile emotion. So can keeping an anger journal, where you write about your feelings and how the disease makes you mad.

Low-impact exercise such as walking or swimming can help your body release some of the anger you hold inside. Discuss with your doctor an appropriate type of exercise program and then stick with it so that you continue to reap its physical and emotional benefits.

Using your creativity to express your frustrations and anger can be greatly freeing.

"Explore creative outlets for anger," says Waldman. "For example, paint, using angry colors like red and orange, even if you don't consider yourself to be an artist."

Besides the visual arts, music can often unlock the less tangible aspects of anger, the raw emotion underpinning your rage. Singing, playing an instrument, or surrounding yourself with music can be a cathartic and inspiring pursuit.

Once you have acknowledged and defined your anger, focus on taking positive action. By doing this, you will spend less time and energy being consumed by your anger and move toward accepting yourself and your life with lupus. Some positive activities include volunteering for a nonprofit organization, becoming a leader in a lupus support group, or tutoring someone in need of extra academic help. By reaching out in these or other ways, you can give yourself a sense of usefulness and worth that can ease the anger you feel within. Making a positive difference in your community is an excellent way to improve your well-being, and that of the world around you, too.

If you find anger taking hold of your life, talk to a professional counselor about ways in which you can channel your anger into something positive. Whatever you do, don't let the anger eat away at you! Acknowledge it, accept it, and use it to fuel your energies to build a more meaningful life.

Fear

Fear and its cousin, anxiety, are very common, very real emotions that lupus patients and their loved ones feel. There is fear of the unknown, of how lupus will affect the patient, and if or how it will progress. There is fear of the financial burden of coping with a chronic illness. In many cases, there is fear that life will be fraught with pain and sorrow. Often, lupus patients fear death.

Coping with Fear

Just as with denial and anger, you need to acknowledge and accept your fear before you can move through it. For many lupus patients, this is difficult because fear can be equated with weakness or "wimpiness"; it can be viewed as the opposite of what today's society expects from strong, "modern" women and men. Very few people today, lupus patients or others, want to admit that they are afraid.

The truth is that by acknowledging your fear, you are being strong and taking charge of it and your disease. By accepting it, you are moving forward to accepting lupus and achieving your desired quality of life.

"Tackling fear and anxiety means taking steps to regain a sense of control over your life," says Lisa Waldman. "It means breaking each fear down into bite-sized chunks, exploring each one in detail. It means doing research, reading books, and talking to other patients and professionals so that you can make appropriate decisions in your life."

The first thing you need to do to cope with your fear is to delve deep inside yourself to discover just what it is you're afraid of. Is it financial trouble? Broken relationships? Loss of self-image? Disability? Loss of cherished goals and dreams?

Once you have determined what it is you are afraid of, articulate your specific fear. Write about it in your lupus diary. Talk to a trusted loved one, saying, "I'm afraid of _____." Ask for your loved one's support and guidance as you search for ways to take charge of your specific fear.

Learn all you can about the options available to you for overcoming your fear. If you are afraid of financial difficulties, consult with a local consumer credit counseling service or certified public accountant (CPA). Look into ways to better budget your finances and plan for rainy days.

If you are afraid of becoming unattractive to yourself and others because of weight gain, hair loss, rashes, and other visible signs of lupus and medication side effects, explore positive ways that you can enhance your body image through exercise, makeup, and wardrobe.

If you are afraid of disability, research and try out ways that you can work around your disability. New household gadgets make cooking and housekeeping easier for persons with arthritic hands. Activities such as travel and attending public events can be easier if you avail yourself of services available to people with disabilities.

Before you were diagnosed with lupus, you may have had a tendency to act independently, to rely on yourself to accomplish your goals. For someone used to a high degree of independence, having lupus and giving in to pain and other debilitating symptoms can be terrifying.

For your own well-being, you must learn the skill of when and how to ask others for help. True friends and caring loved ones will welcome the chance to assist you in cooking, driving, or just listening, but you have to be willing to ask. Look upon asking for help as a way to take charge of your disease. See your reliance upon others as a wonderful gift and take (and give) joy in knowing you are appreciated and loved.

Take your fear to a lupus support group and ask other patients how they have handled the same situations and fears. This will help you with specific problems and also enable you to feel that you're not alone.

Certainly, rely on your faith to bolster your courage in facing your fears and overcoming them. Prayer, meditation, positive affirmation, and a supportive faith community can bring tremendous comfort and insight to your troubled soul, heart, and body. The constancy of religious ritual can also be calming when everything else in your life seems up in the air.

Of all your fears, perhaps fear of the unknown is the most difficult one to cope with. The course of lupus is unpredictable, and you cannot control how and what others feel about the disease, nor can you control how they react to you. In all your searching, be honest with yourself. What are the aspects of your fear that you can control? What do you need to let go of? Continue to ask yourself these questions and listen carefully and patiently for the answers. Take steps to address those things that you have control over so that they are no longer worrisome to you. Try not to hold on to things over which you have no control.

Fear of Death

For many lupus patients, the fear of death is the most terrifying of all. Fortunately, fewer lupus patients die from the disease than ever before. New treatments, earlier diagnoses, and a better understanding of the intricacies of the illness make it possible for physicians to control the symptoms and, many times, the disease progression. As research continues, and more information unfolds about the nature of autoimmune diseases, there is every reason to hope that the future is even brighter than the present when it comes to lupus prognoses.

But you will still hear the stories of people who know people who died from lupus. And much of the media coverage focuses on the debilitating aspects of the disease. It is no wonder that you and your loved ones should feel fear.

Talking with your doctor about your specific prognosis can help you put your fear of death into perspective. Keeping your mind and heart focused on living will also take the edge of darkness off of your days and nights. Exploring with a trained counselor or clergyperson how you feel about death can demystify some of your fear.

Faith can be tremendously uplifting when fears of death seem to overwhelm you. Knowing that there is a constant, eternal presence beyond yourself can help you know that you are never alone, never unloved, and thus never need to despair.

Sorrow

Sorrow is an emotion shared by many lupus patients. It springs from a sense of loss of health, of life as they knew it, as well as frustration at knowing that there is no cure for lupus, no light at the end of the tunnel. Sorrow may come and go as your disease ebbs and flows, but at times it might seem all-encompassing and never-ending.

Just as with anger and denial, you want to make sure that you do not rest in the sorrow for an extended period of time.

Coping with Sorrow

To lessen the burden of sorrow, find a way to express it so that you do not hold it inside for long. Share your fears and your vulnerability with a loved one or your lupus support group. Cry, if you feel like it. There is nothing wrong with crying, nor is there anything wrong with laughing, which can be a natural reaction, too, during times of deep sorrow.

Write about your sadness in your lupus diary, being blunt about your negative emotions. Seek counseling, especially if you feel you might be slipping from sorrow into depression, which happens to many lupus patients.

With lupus, your body is at war with itself. Being kind to yourself is key to successfully coping with lupus. When you feel yourself dragging or becoming sad, do something nice for yourself. I know

Lupus and Depression

There is some evidence that the stress response in patients who are predisposed to autoimmune diseases such as lupus is impaired so that there is a decrease in the production of steroid-releasing hormones. This can predispose a patient to the development of a melancholic type of depression that impairs the person's ability to cope with pain and disability. In fact, most lupus patients do experience depression at some point during the course of their illness. Treatment of depression can improve one's sense of mastery over one's illness.

Denial of the severity of an illness and belief that alternative forms of treatment may heal a chronic illness such as lupus are unfortunately self-destructive ways of coping with any incurable illness. Working with a therapist can help one suppress thoughts of disbelief and denial that occur and face the challenges that living with lupus can bring.

this might sound simplistic, but it is very important. Sometimes taking a walk, buying yourself flowers, watching a funny movie, or taking special care with clothing or jewelry can lift the spirits just enough to make a positive difference.

In times of sorrow and pain, your faith is a vital support for you. Prayer and meditation can ease the burden of grief you feel, even sometimes lowering your blood pressure and helping your whole body to physically calm down. Keep a collection of uplifting Scripture verses or other inspirational writing, and quietly allow yourself to take time with the soothing words of others. Take inspiration from the stories of others who have suffered great hardships and overcome them.

By flooding your soul with affirming thoughts and prayers you can fill yourself with love and comfort, easing even your deepest sorrow.

Guilt

"If only I hadn't . . ."

When they are diagnosed, many lupus patients ask their doctors and themselves what they could have done to prevent getting their disease. You, too, might have asked whether your vacation in the sun, brand of hair coloring, or stressful divorce made you get lupus. You might feel guilty that you brought on the disease, and this guilt might make you angry and afraid to take positive steps to help yourself medically, socially, or spiritually.

On the other hand, you might blame another person, a parent, perhaps, for giving you "bad genes," or a boss for making you so stressed you got sick. Your loved ones, too, might feel guilty that they did something to bring on your lupus. This guilt can put a wedge between you and those you need to help you cope with your disease.

Guilt can create high degrees of internal stress. It is detrimental to finding a good quality of life with lupus. You need to address it definitively.

Coping with Guilt

Learning all you can about the causes of lupus will help you rid yourself of unnecessary guilt. First, understand that lupus is not contagious; you cannot get it from another person, and you cannot give it to someone else now that you have it.

There are probably complex genetic and environmental components that go into lupus's development, so you can't blame yourself or another person for individual activities or genes that caused you to develop it.

Lupus can flare even if you follow all of your doctor's orders. Of course, you need to take all your medications and refrain from activities that are known to exacerbate lupus or bring on flares, such as prolonged exposure to the sun or allowing yourself to be in extremely stressful situations. But sometimes a lupus flare will just happen, and you cannot feel guilty because of it.

Reassurance from your doctor and loved ones will help you overcome your guilt. Expressing it aloud will also help you understand that there are some things out of your control. You did nothing wrong to get lupus. Just accept that sometimes, lupus simply is.

Acceptance

Each of your many emotions helps you to move through your grieving process toward acceptance of your new life with lupus. This acceptance will not happen all at once, nor will it always be easy. You may resist it at times, and cover yourself in denial. You may rage at lupus. You may feel sorrow, fear, and guilt.

But ultimately, taking charge of lupus means accepting your life with the disease. Because there is no cure for lupus, you must accept the fact that you will have to live with a chronic illness, one for which there is no end in sight.

The Benefits of Acceptance

When you accept lupus, you are able to take productive steps toward seeking appropriate medical care and making lifestyle changes that augment your health, inside and out. You can achieve a new level of honesty and insight with your relationships with loved ones, and you can experience greater degrees of love and joy in those relationships and the new ones that you forge because of the opportunities lupus will bring to you.

Knowing that you have lupus will make you more able to understand the suffering of others and could lead you to become a more compassionate person. You might engage in volunteer opportunities because of this increased empathy, and through your work, you could make a significant difference in the world around you.

You might discover new work that brings you fulfillment. You might rediscover the joy of just living, just *being* in the midst of a hectic, noisy world.

Acceptance of your lupus and your ability to cope with it will increase your faith by leaps and bounds. You will find strength you didn't know you had and abilities you were unaware of.

By accepting lupus, you will be able to take positive steps to strengthen yourself and your relationships with others. You will find that, although your life is changed, it is by no means over.

You Are Not a Wimp!

As you cope with the many changes that lupus brings, you might find yourself thinking that you are weak, escaping from life, or copping out.

Of course, you want to make sure that you do not use lupus as an excuse not to live up to your responsibilities. You still need to see that your finances and other personal obligations are tended to. If you have children, you cannot stop being a parent. If you decide to keep working, you cannot suddenly cease performing your job.

But the fatigue, pain, and uncertainty that lupus brings will, at times, weigh you down. There will be days when you cannot go outdoors, or cannot work or cook or clean house. You could lose productivity, physical capabilities, even the appearance you once had. You might begin to feel useless and insignificant. Your self-esteem might plummet.

Unfortunately, these emotions are common among lupus patients. But the patients who cope successfully with the disease do not let themselves get weighed down by them for very long. Acknowledge how you are feeling, and then realize that flares can be treated. Time, patience, and perseverance can heal much of the discomfort and anguish caused by lupus.

5

THE MEDICAL FACTOR:

What You Can Do

Many newly diagnosed lupus patients are bewildered at the sudden role that medications and medical personnel play in their lives. Regular doctor visits, tests, and treatments seem to suddenly take over a once-healthy life. And, unlike with most nonchronic illnesses, with lupus the stream of appointments, retests, and refills seems to never end.

In fact, as long as there is no cure for lupus, these medical components will always be a part of the lupus patient's life. Keeping on top of your medical condition is imperative to maintaining your health. Ignoring the crucial role of medicine in your life could lead to disaster.

Health

You cannot achieve any other goal until you have a firm handle on how you need to take care of yourself. It usually takes two to three years after diagnosis for a patient to have a good sense of what symptoms are particular to his or her lupus. So although your top priority might be watching out for your health (as it should be), what this means in practical terms will take several years to unfold—and then lupus can still surprise you, even ten or twenty years later!

This does not mean that you have to give up planning anything else, and it does not mean that there won't be time for your other goals and dreams to become realities. It means you will have to accept being flexible in the face of flares and ready to communicate your health needs as they arise, rather than trying to sweep them under the rug so that you can appear to be productive or super-strong.

Denial, Denial

When you are bombarded with instructions about things you can and cannot do, medication regimens, and medical tests and examination schedules, your first impulse might be to try to squeeze them in, to try to continue on your normal life without giving in to your weakened health. This is a natural reaction, and hearkens back to the sense of denial that all new lupus patients have, to one degree or another. However, lupus is not like getting a cold or other virus that will run its course. Lupus is a disease that cannot be ignored. If left unchecked, its course can cause you permanent damage or, in the worst instance, death. Face your denial head-on, acknowledging that it exists. Then do what you need to follow your doctor's orders and start yourself on the road to harnessing your symptoms and arresting your flare.

A Delicate Balance

Sometimes you will get conflicting information about how to proceed with an aspect of your lupus treatment. Because autoimmune diseases can be difficult to fully understand, doctors might not agree on what you can do about a particular problem. In this case, you need to be the arbiter, gathering as much information from all sides as you can. You need to discuss the situation thoroughly with your rheumatologist and, ultimately, rely on the solution that you and he or she feel will be most likely to handle the problem.

When There Is No Answer

Lupus can manifest itself in a myriad of different ways. In some rare instances, there might be no clear treatment for a particular problem. Then you will have to accept it when your doctor says, "There's really nothing we can do." Understand that there might not be an answer now, but there could be in the future. Live as best you can with the discomfort, but do not let it lead you to a depression. Hope and have faith that someday there *will* be something that can be done.

Humor as a Tool

A sense of humor is a tool of choice among many lupus patients who battle severe and mild disease. One lupus patient develops stand-up comedy routines and delivers them regularly. Another collects funny frog statues, pictures, and stories and turns to them for comic relief. Another still has adopted three cats that are forever amusing her.

If you do not know what tickles your funny bone, now is the time to find out. Explore the comics, the humor section of the bookstore, the curio section of an antique store—find something that makes you smile and use it regularly and liberally to brighten your mood when the pain is at its worst. Also, surrounding yourself with people who make you smile and laugh will help bring you out of the pain, too. Laughter is, to be sure, a potent medicine!

Your Role

As a lupus patient, you will see doctors, nurses, lab technicians, and a host of other medical professionals. However, the ultimate responsibility for your health rests upon you. Here are some of the things that you should do as a responsible lupus patient:

- Keep scrupulous track of your doctor appointments, scheduling them as you would meetings for your job.

- Be on time for your doctor appointments, and bring all the necessary paperwork/notes/questions.
- Take all prescribed medication as directed by your physician.
- Notify your physician of any and all side effects or other concerns stemming from your medication.
- Be conscientious about not engaging in activities that might aggravate your lupus. This includes avoiding prolonged exposure to the sun, wearing appropriate sun-protective attire and sunblock if you need to go outside, and staying out of situations where you could be exposed to infection or stress of the joints.
- Keep abreast of the latest developments in lupus research, treatment, and medications. Discuss these with your doctor.
- Do not participate in diets or alternative treatments unless you have discussed them thoroughly with your doctor and he or she agrees that you can go ahead.
- Keep up-to-date on all other medical appointments, including regular dental, eye, and gynecological checkups. Report any irregularities to your rheumatologist.
- Know what your health plan covers and keep current on the status of insurance reimbursement and doctors' bills.

First Things First

Upon receiving your diagnosis, talk with your doctor about what lifestyle changes you need to make in order to lessen the harmful medical effects of lupus. If you are in a severe flare, it might not be prudent for you to work, at least as long as it takes to get the flare under control. If you choose to continue working, you might need to modify your work hours or reduce them significantly. Or you might need to change your profession if you perform work that puts you in harm's way (a job where you work in the sun, for example, if you are sun sensitive).

Discuss all medications and possible side effects and find out exactly how much and when you need to take medications. Determine whether you will need to alter your eating habits because of your medications (for example, limiting alcohol intake). Know what to do if you accidentally skip a dose.

If you suffer from joint pain, your current exercise regimen might be too strenuous for you. Ask your doctor about how to develop an exercise program that can work for you—and change your schedule to stick with it!

Some of your future plans might have to be changed, too. It might not be prudent for you to travel if you are fighting a flare, or you might need to rearrange your itinerary so that you can get in the necessary rest to keep your body going. Taking on the leadership role in a charitable event or organization might be too much of a burden for you right now. Starting a new job might also be too stressful for you, as could beginning a new course of study.

As you discuss what you should not do, determine what you can do instead. Deal with the losses in your life as ways to develop new activities, interests, and people. Keep in mind that the progression of lupus is very difficult to determine, and you might find yourself changing direction more than once along the way. Look upon a life with lupus as an adventure that will yield some good with the difficult. You will find yourself responding in a much more productive, positive way.

Pain Management

Besides the emotional upheaval caused by a diagnosis of lupus, there is physical pain associated with the disease, the tests, and the treatments used to combat it. Of course, different patients experience different degrees of physical pain. Sometimes it is minor (a pinprick to give blood for tests). Sometimes it might be excruciating (joint pain that renders you unable to walk). But always, the pain is discomforting and reminds you that you are ill.

Things to Do to Manage Pain

➤ Talk with your doctor about the source of your pain and what, if any, medical steps can be taken to alleviate it.
➤ Work with a physical or occupational therapist to enable you to move and work more comfortably.
➤ Ask your pharmacist for tips on coping with the side effects of your medication, especially chemotherapy drugs.
➤ Consult with a counselor or clergyperson to help you cope with the emotional toll pain can take.

➤ *Learn deep-breathing techniques and use them when pain begins.*

➤ *Pray and meditate, using positive affirmations to counteract the negative effects of pain.*

➤ *Read, listen to music, practice a craft, or play with a pet to distract your mind from your pain.*

➤ *Talk to a friend and articulate your pain to them.*

➤ *Observe nature to remind yourself that there is a world beyond the internal pain that you feel.*

Some Tips on Giving Blood

Many tests used to determine the extent of lupus activity are conducted by taking samples of blood and then analyzing them. As a lupus patient, you will often be asked to give multiple blood samples. Here are some tips on making the blood-giving process a little less painful:

- Breathe in deeply just as the lab technician inserts the needle to begin drawing blood.
- Look away instead of directly at the vials as they are filling.
- Ask for a "butterfly" needle, which is thinner and will not put as much stress on your veins.
- Think of a pleasant place or activity as you have your blood drawn.

How to Cope with Side Effects of Medications Such as Prednisone, Antimalarial Medications, or Chemotherapy

Side effects of medications may often be identified as new symptoms of lupus. Prednisone is a medicine used to treat various manifestations of lupus, from kidney or brain involvement, to stubborn rashes, to severe fatigue. Yet the medication can often cause mood swings, depression, and skin problems resulting in bruises and reddish rashes due to new blood vessels forming in the skin. If this medication is tapered abruptly and stopped, it usually leads to widespread pain and fatigue. This leads to an unending cycle of steroid dependence, which can lead to well-known complications of steroids such as brittle bones, high blood pressure, and high blood sugars.

An astute rheumatologist or an informed patient will recognize the pain and fatigue to be steroid withdrawal and fibromyalgia and will take appropriate steps to prevent it or treat the symptoms till they are resolved. Although prednisone is a miraculous medication and improves symptoms and prevents organ damage in lupus patients, the duration of therapy with it must be short (a few weeks for non-organ-threatening lupus and three to six months for organ-threatening manifestations). I advocate the aggressive use of prednisone-sparing drugs such as azathioprine (Imuran) and hydroxychloroquine (Plaquenil) to limit the duration of prednisone use. Some muscle relaxants and sleep aids can help with the steroid withdrawal symptoms, and specific treatments for depression and osteoporosis can be added on if needed to counter these side effects.

Antimalarial drugs such as hydroxychloroquine can lead to itchy rashes due to an allergic reaction in the first few weeks and a bluish-black pigment deposition in the shins and mucous membranes after years of use. These must be differentiated from complications of lupus before appropriate treatments can be determined.

Medicines such as methotrexate and azathioprine, which are used to treat cancer in high doses, are often used in low doses to treat organ-threatening manifestations of lupus such as kidney disease. Predictable side effects such as nausea, loss of appetite, and infections can be prevented or treated expeditiously if they should occur. Nausea due to these medications tends to occur only on the day of administration, which is once a week in the case of methotrexate, and can be countered with antinausea medications. Infections may be prevented with vaccinations such as the pneumococcal vaccine. Four different prescription medications may be used to abbreviate the flu, since the use of the flu vaccine in lupus can result in lupus flares in certain lupus subsets.

Do Patients with Lupus Need to Take Medications Throughout Their Lives? When Does One Decide When to Stop Taking Medication?

Since a cure for lupus eludes us for now, medications and therapies have to be tailored to the symptoms and manifestations in individual patients. It is possible to induce a remission of symptoms of joint pain and fatigue with medications such as hydroxychloroquine or low doses of methotrexate, a chemotherapy medication. More serious organ involvement such as kidney disease can also be pushed into inactivity by using monthly intravenous pulse doses of cyclophosphamide for six months.

Once a remission of symptoms is achieved, it is prudent to maintain remission with maintenance regimens such as thrice-weekly hydroxychloroquine for non-organ-threatening illness and immunosuppressive drugs such as azathioprine (Imuran) for organ involvement for a period of two or more years. Lupus may "burn itself out" over fifteen to twenty years provided all activity is adequately suppressed. Many patients need only annual or biannual surveillance at this point. Only careful monitoring of symptoms, signs, and laboratory tests can enable you to safely come off medications.

6

THE MEDICAL FACTOR:

Your Lupus
Medical Team

During the course of your life with lupus, you will encounter many health-care professionals. Putting together your medical team and working with the various members of it is one of the most important aspects of coping with lupus. You begin by identifying whom you need to include on your team and what role each member will play in managing your health care.

Who's Who

Although lupus is an autoimmune disease, patients come to their diagnoses through many different medical channels. Some are diagnosed by a **general practitioner** (G.P., or **internal medicine** specialist). Others are first tested by a **dermatologist** (a doctor who treats diseases of the skin), **ophthalmologist** (who treats the eye), **dentist** (who treats the mouth and teeth), or other medical professional.

The key medical specialist who is trained and certified to identify and treat autoimmune diseases is a **rheumatologist.** This individual is a Doctor of Medicine (M.D.) with a specialty in internal medicine and a subspecialty in rheumatology. There were approximately four thousand certified rheumatologists practicing in the United States in 2000.

Depending on a patient's symptoms, the rheumatologist might seek the advice of a number of other medical professionals during the course of your treatment. For example, a **nephrologist** might be called in for problems dealing with the kidneys; a **pulmonologist** for the lungs; a **cardiologist** for the heart; a **gastroenterologist** for the gastrointestinal (GI) tract; or a **neuro-ophthalmologist** for problems involving the nerves of the eye. A **clinical psychologist** or a **psychiatrist** might be called in to help with a patient's emotional health. And a **physical therapist** or **occupational therapist** could be prescribed for exercise and joint-mobility matters.

In some cases, specialists will have subspecialties. For example, an **occupational therapist** might focus on mobility issues concerning the hands (a hand therapist), or a **physical therapist** might specialize in aquatic exercise (pool therapy). Your rheumatologist can direct you to the proper person to treat your specific symptoms. Your support group can also be a source of referral for some hard-to-find specialists.

Another key player on your lupus team is your **pharmacist**. As soon as you have your first prescriptions, you should select a pharmacist in your area and bring all your refills and new prescriptions to him or her. With your complete medication schedule on record, the pharmacist can flag drug interactions and inform you of side effects and dosage instructions. He or she can also help you if you lose your medication or need an emergency refill.

The best kind of pharmacist is one who will take the time to explain your medication to you and listen to your concerns about side effects. He or she should be willing to call your physician if questions arise, or if you need refills. Your pharmacist should also keep meticulous records of your past and current medications in order to inform you of potential drug interactions, should the need arise.

Choosing a Doctor

As you begin your search for a rheumatologist, gather several names, if you can. Ask the other lupus patients you know about their doctors. Find out from them how the doctors relate to them, and if they are satisfied with the level of care they receive. Ask for a referral from your family doctor or other medical professional whom you trust.

There are several databases available on the Internet that can provide you with background information. One of these is the

American Medical Association's Web site. Here you can find out where your doctor went to medical school, when he or she graduated, and what his or her areas of specialty are. Some states keep similar databases; some even provide information about license status and any complaints that have been filed.

The Lupus Foundation of America can provide you with a list of physicians specializing in lupus. The American College of Rheumatology (www.rheumatology.org) keeps a database of certified rheumatologists sorted by geographic area. The American Medical Association (www.ama.org) also has a database of doctors according to specialty.

Once you have gathered your list, you are ready to make your personal assessment of which doctor is right for you. Because you will be working most closely with your primary doctor (usually your rheumatologist), it is important that you feel comfortable with that doctor. This does not mean that your rheumatologist becomes your best friend. But it does mean that you should feel free to communi-

The Essential Role of a Rheumatologist as Part of Your Treatment Team

When a medical student graduates from medical school, he or she decides whether to pursue a career in performing surgery or training for three or more years to become an internist who is an expert in managing diseases of adult men or women. At this stage, there is an overall understanding of the symptoms and signs and treatment of lupus from observing and treating dozens of patients with varying degrees of disease severity.

Internists pursuing a career in rheumatology observe and treat scores of lupus patients during their two years of fellowship training and are thus ideally suited as consultants for this illness. A rheumatologist is the ideal person to be your primary-care provider, and most also serve as the manager of the lupus patient's treatment team, which may include a gynecologist, kidney specialist, skin specialist, transplant specialist, physical therapist, and sometimes an additional internist.

cate your symptoms, concerns, and problems to him or her—and even ask "stupid" questions on occasion.

Assessing a New Physician

When you meet with a rheumatologist for the first time, he or she should do a very thorough physical examination and take a detailed medical history. This is your chance, too, to find out about the rheumatologist. You should:

- Ask questions about his or her training, practice, and expertise in working with lupus patients.
- Observe how he or she talks with you and whether his or her questions to you sound genuinely caring.
- Feel comfortable asking questions and confident that the answers you receive are thoughtful and not hurried or condescending.

Another important aspect of choosing your physician is the way in which he or she runs the practice and staffs the office. Your doctor's office should be:

- Clean and well organized.
- Well staffed, with at least one nurse on hand and an attentive, caring receptionist.
- A pleasant place, with no undercurrent of stress and/or anger.
- Efficiently run so that you do not have to wait a long time past your scheduled appointment before being seen by the doctor (unless there is an unforeseen medical emergency).

Gather Information

Be sure to find out and note your doctor's office hours, telephone hours, and what to do if an emergency occurs after hours. Ask about the procedure for putting through insurance claims and payment schedules. Find out where lab work is processed, how long it takes to complete it, and the way in which the doctor will communicate results to you. Some patients do not like to wait until their next appointment and would rather speak with the doctor about the tests as soon as the results are known, even if the results are normal. (Of course, your doctor should notify you immediately of any irregularities in your tests.)

Trust Your Instincts

Once you have all these questions answered, you will need to take a more subjective pulse of how you feel you interact with the doctor. The most brilliant physician in the world might not be a good match for you if you do not feel comfortable speaking with him or her. Likewise, if you find that the doctor is too familiar with you, or does not have enough expertise in an area that pertains to your case of lupus, you might not feel assurance about his or her ability to treat you effectively. No doctor is perfect; but you should choose the one who will be the best fit with you *and* your medical condition.

Communicating with Your Doctor

You should feel comfortable asking your doctor any and every question pertaining to your health. However, you need to convey those questions in an appropriate, responsible manner. The key to getting your questions answered satisfactorily is to be well prepared.

Prepare Your Questions in Advance

Before you go to your doctor appointment, write down all your questions, as well as your current medications and dosages, on a sheet of paper. Make a copy for yourself and give the original to

---

What You Should Expect from Your Doctor

All lupus patients should strive to find doctors who are knowledgeable and who will return their telephone messages on the same day that they call. Although many of the issues that lupus patients experience may not seem unique for the physician, it is very important that the patient's complaints are heard by the doctor and not brushed away.

It is critical to develop long-term relationships with your providers, but do not feel shy or insecure about seeking a second opinion regarding a specific aspect of your condition. A good doctor will not feel threatened by your desire to help yourself and should not take offense if it is done openly.

your doctor. Writing your questions in advance allows you to be thoughtful and to articulate your concerns. It also makes sure that you don't forget anything. Besides your prescribed medications, include any herbal supplements or over-the-counter preparations that you have taken since your last visit or are currently taking. It's a good idea to bring the bottle or box with the list of ingredients, especially for herbal or homeopathic substances, in case your doctor wants to study it.

When you formulate your questions, try to be as articulate as possible. For example, instead of writing, *What about the pain?* be specific: *What can I do for my knee spasms?* Include the frequency (number of times, time of day) with which the discomfort or symptom occurs, and any other information you can give that will give your doctor an ample picture of how to proceed (whether the pain comes after doing a certain exercise, for example).

Sometimes consulting a thesaurus will help you choose the correct words to use in describing a type of pain or rash. Don't be afraid to use analogies, either! Saying, "My head feels like there's a bass drum playing a solo" gives your physician a more vivid picture of the type of headache you could be experiencing than if you said only, "My head hurts."

Take Notes

When you discuss your questions with your doctor, write down his or her responses on your copy of the question sheet. Make a clear notation about any medications, or changes in medications, that he or she prescribes. Bring your calendar and note the specific days that correspond with dosages to be taken and when to begin tapering off.

Taking notes during an appointment will save you a lot of wondering later!

In addition to your current questions, keep a log of all the symptoms that have occurred since your last visit, including the type, frequency, and time of day (see Sample Symptom Log, pages 67–68). Bring this log to your office visit and discuss it with your doctor. Your physician can help you put together a pattern that might point to an underlying autoimmune problem. When you are first diagnosed, it's typical to ignore some symptoms as insignificant. For example, if you awaken in the morning and find your tongue stuck to the roof of your mouth frequently, this could be an indication of a drug side effect or perhaps Sjögren's syndrome. By writing down everything, you might find many of the symptoms do not require serious consideration. But in those rare cases when you are able to identify something that needs treatment, you will be better off.

Take Charge of Your Medical Records

In addition to providing you with medical care, your rheumatologist is your first line of communication to and among the specialists who will deal with various aspects of your disease or overall health. You should request that a copy of all medical reports be sent to your rheumatologist, who should keep the most comprehensive medical file on your condition. This includes your regular dental, eye, and gynecological checkups (which you should still keep up with, even if you are under the regular care of a rheumatologist).

Whenever you go to a specialist (not your regular lupus doctor), bring a copy of your list of current medications, and your symptom log. It is also an excellent idea to keep a "medical résumé" (see sample, page 62) and attach it to the form that you need to fill out when first visiting the specialist. This will save you from having to write out your medical history again and again, as well as provide an updated, clear record of your health for the physician who is not familiar with you at all.

TIP: Practice Diplomatic Assertiveness

If you feel intimidated by your doctor, but also feel that you are not receiving the kind of medical care you feel you need, try to practice "diplomatic assertiveness" before you give up on that doctor altogether.

Lisa Waldman, licensed clinical psychotherapist and health educator, says, "This technique involves overcoming feelings of intimidation, which are inherent in the doctor/patient relationship because of the power differential. It means asking for the time, the information, and the listening ear that you need in a respectful and calm manner that demonstrates both your awareness of your doctor's circumstances as well as your own rights and needs as a patient."

Other Things Your Doctor Might Do

At some point in your life with lupus, you might become disabled. Accompanying the disability will be paperwork required by the government agency or private insurance company handling your claim. Your doctor will need to fill out part of the forms, and usually the time frame for doing so is crucial to getting your claim considered.

When it comes to filling out disability forms and other paperwork, be sure to give your physician enough time to complete the necessary information. Needing something "yesterday" not only causes stress for you, but it makes life more frenzied for your physician. Be considerate, and make life easier for both of you.

When Your Doctor Is Not Available

Because of the chronic, ongoing nature of the disease, the relationship between a lupus doctor and his or her patient can become a close one. Still, understand that your doctor might not be available when you call. Leave a number where you can be reached, and a time frame during which you will be at that number. Most physicians try to return telephone calls within twenty-four hours. If you find that your doctor does not return your calls, or is severely delayed in doing so, express your concern with your physician and ask if there is a better way to get a more prompt response (some doctors rely on e-mail to communicate with patients, too).

If you have a true emergency, expect prompt attention! Your doctor should have an after-hours answering service and there should be a physician on call, available through that service, at all times. Do not expect your doctor to be on call every night, but do expect that there will be a competent doctor available in case of emergency. If there is not, you should probably look for another lupus doctor—lupus is a disease that can flare at any time, and you need to be covered appropriately.

What Symptoms Constitute a True Emergency in a Lupus Patient

Symptoms such as seizures, alteration in mental status, swelling of the legs, severe shortness of breath, chest pain, bleeding or easy bruising, or persistent high fevers may signal organ involvement in lupus and constitute an emergency. Lupus patients may be hospitalized in the first year of their illness if they have involvement of their blood cells, kidney, heart, brain, or lungs.

Sometimes the presentation of lupus is with a seizure due to brain involvement or due to fluid accumulating around the heart. This is a catastrophic presentation and usually requires hospitalization for intravenous steroids and close monitoring.

When a new medication is started by your doctor, ask your doctor what you can expect in terms of benefits from the medication and what side effects you need to watch for. Side effects such as swelling of the lips or throat or severe rashes could be dangerous if ignored and must be reported to your doctor immediately.

If You Don't Get Along with Your Doctor

Voicing Complaints

If you have a complaint about the way in which your doctor is treating you, do not let it fester. First, try to clear the air by calmly discussing your concern(s) with your doctor and offering solutions. For example, if he or she allows frequent interruptions during your office visit, request that your next appointment be scheduled at a time when there will be no (or far fewer) interruptions.

If you have a personality conflict with your doctor, first try to determine whether it comes from a true clash or from a conflict between you and your disease. Internal frustration at not being cured can sometimes be displaced, directed at the physician who treats you. In cases such as this, it is a good idea to seek professional counseling so that you can achieve a better level of coping and working with your doctor.

Sometimes, however, even after a careful selection process, you and your physician might have a falling-out. Your health is the most important thing to think about. It is better to go on to another, more compatible doctor than to jeopardize your health by continuing to work with one whom you do not trust.

Changing Doctors

There are many reasons why patients change doctors. Sometimes the physicians retire, move, or pare back their practices. Sometimes patients move to another city or become dissatisfied with their current care. Still other times, a physician might determine that the patient's symptoms are such that another physician with a different specialty might better handle them.

Moving On

Although your physician is not your best friend, moving on to another might be traumatic if you have had a good working relationship throughout your treatment. You should acknowledge that you need to go through a modified period of mourning, but do not let that interfere with your ability to work with your new physician. Still, no two doctors practice medicine in the same manner, so give yourself and your new doctor a chance to adjust.

If you are moving and need to find a new rheumatologist, you should:

- Ask your current doctor for a referral, if appropriate.
- Ask yourself why, if you are dissatisfied with the level of care you receive from your current physician. Do you believe that he or she is not doing everything possible to treat you, or is giving you inadequate care? Do you have an expectation of finding the "perfect cure"? Or do you not want to take medication at all and hope to find a doctor who will tell you that you do not need to?
- Carefully assess your reasons for wanting to change doctors. Follow the procedure outlined above for choosing a doctor.
- If you feel it necessary, discuss with your previous doctor the reason for your change in as objective a manner as possible.

- Obtain a copy of all records kept by your former physician. This includes lab work, physician's notes, and any forms that were filled out or filed. Arrange these notes/files in chronological order, make a copy for yourself, and pass the originals along to your new physician.
- Tell your loved ones about your switch in physicians. Also, tell the specialists with whom you consult about the change and the new address to which they should send their reports.
- Update your telephone number list and any medical alert tags you wear.
- If you left your doctor because you did not get along, be careful how you explain what you did to other lupus patients. Perhaps your personalities did not mesh, but that

Information to Include on Your Medical Résumé

NAME
ADDRESS
PHONE NUMBER
SOCIAL SECURITY NUMBER
EMERGENCY CONTACT
PHYSICIAN/ADDRESS/TELEPHONE NUMBER
INSURANCE CARRIER/ADDRESS

CURRENT MEDICAL CONDITIONS
CURRENT MEDICATIONS/DOSAGES
DATE OF LAST CHEST X RAY
DATE OF LAST CARDIAC WORKUP (What was done?)
DATE OF LAST GYNECOLOGICAL EXAM
DATE OF LAST MAMMOGRAM

HOSPITALIZATION HISTORY:
    Where, When, Why, Attending Physician
SURGERY HISTORY:
    Where, When, Why, Attending Physician

does not mean that the physician will not be effective for someone else. There is a subjective side to choosing a doctor, and each lupus patient should respect another patient's choice, as long as the medical care provided is effective and appropriate.

Switching from "Western Medicine" to Alternatives

At this time, there is no effective, overall lupus treatment available that is completely alternative in scope. Some forms of alternative treatments can be helpful in treating some of the symptoms of lupus. For example, acupuncture can alleviate some of the pain, and massage can establish a better sense of well-being. But it is still a prudent idea to seek out alternative therapies with your rheumatologist's guidance and approval.

7

THE MEDICAL FACTOR:

Record Keeping
Made Easier

The first time you see a doctor, you have to fill out forms. When you submit claims to your insurance company, you have to fill out forms. Having your health information handy for your doctor visits and insurance company will save you much time and aggravation. It will also ease your worry when lupus fog takes hold and you can't quite remember the right names or numbers!

The Forms Others Give You to Fill Out

At the time you make an appointment to see a doctor for the first time, ask if you can receive a copy of any paperwork you need to fill out in advance of your meeting. If this is impossible, have a medical or health history résumé handy to attach to the paperwork you will get at the doctor's office. Also have a separate form with your insurance numbers, contact names and telephone numbers, and any other pertinent information the doctor needs. As discussed in the previous chapter, when you go for your office visit, have two pieces of paper handy to give to your doctor: one with your current list of medications, complete with dosages, the other with your list of current symptoms and questions.

TIP: Fill Out Forms When Your Hands Are Healthy

When your hands are up to it, take a bit of time to complete as much information as you can on several insurance claim forms (write in your name, address, group number, etc.). Leave all the individual claim information blank; you will be able to fill this in when you have an actual claim. Doing this will save you time when you need to fill out the form.

Tracking Symptoms

The reason you need to track your symptoms is so that you and your doctor can determine how best to approach and treat them. Also, figuring out if there is a causal link between one or more symptoms and/or activity/medication/stress factor can help you better manage your lupus and in some cases give you more peace of mind that you are not "falling apart."

Consistency is the most important thing when you track your symptoms. If you use one number or word to denote your pain level one day and change to another word or number the next, you will confuse yourself and whoever else needs to read the information.

The "Value" of Symptoms

Giving a numerical value is probably the easiest way to interpret your level of pain, fatigue, depression, stress, or activity impairment. For example, you can use a scale of 0 to 10, with 0 being no pain/stress/etc., and 10 being the worst. You could also use a smaller scale, say 0 to 3, if you feel that would be easier. But again, be consistent with which scale you use throughout your tracking.

Besides relating the intensity of the pain, impairment, or other symptom, you should try to develop a descriptive vocabulary that can give your physician an idea of what kind of pain, etc., you feel. For example, if you feel a sharp, jabbing pain in your foot, explain it like that, rather than saying, "My foot really hurts."

Another way of describing symptoms that can come in handy is to liken them to other phenomena: "My head felt like I traveled upward in an elevator and then plunged down really quickly."

Choose similar circumstances that are understandable by the average person and be ready to describe the symptom another way if the first way doesn't convey exactly what you mean. Rashes may be difficult to describe, and it may not always be feasible to go in for an appointment when they are visible. Taking pictures of a changing rash can provide a wealth of information to your doctor, especially when rashes last for a short period of time.

How to Communicate Symptoms that Are Difficult to Measure, Such as Lupus Fatigue and Lupus Fog

Some symptoms in lupus such as rashes, hair loss, or kidney disease, are easy to detect by physical examination or by laboratory tests. Other symptoms, such as migraine headaches, depression, lupus fatigue, and mental fogginess, are not readily apparent on examination or by tests.

Keeping a headache diary noting the frequency and severity of headaches helps to monitor response to treatment. A surrogate measure for the severity of fatigue or depression is the number of days missed from work. Loss of work productivity and missing workdays often helps to bring these symptoms to your physician's attention. Another way to measure the severity of lupus fatigue and fog is to rate these symptoms on a scale of 0 to 10, where 10 is the worst score one can imagine.

It is often difficult to admit to being depressed and to relay this to a physician, but ongoing symptoms of feeling blue, crying spells, lack of interest in activities that usually interest us, excessive sleep or lack of sleep, and weight gain or loss often signal depression. Early intervention treats these conditions better than when they become chronic.

A Sampling of Forms

Sample Symptom Summary Log

This log can give a week's worth of symptom levels at a glance. It can also serve to show causal links between certain symptoms, for example between the level of pain and the level of fatigue and/or depression. It is usually used in conjunction with the written symptom log, which gives a more descriptive measure of symptoms and actions taken to treat them.

Sample Symptom Summary Log
Rated 1 to 3

Symptom	Sun	Mon	Tues	Wed	Thurs	Fri	Sat
PAIN	3	3	2	1	1	1	1
FATIGUE	3	3	3	2	2	1	1
DEPRESSION	3	3	3	2	2	2	2
STRESS LEVEL	3	3	3	2	2	2	1
ACTIVITY IMPAIRMENT	1	3	3	2	2	2	2

Symptom Log

This log will take a more "storytelling" view of relating symptoms. Think of it as your lupus symptom diary, complete with your questions and concerns.

Sample Symptom Log
Sunday, August 2
Played with the dog outside in hot sun. Knew I shouldn't have, but I've been so worried about Jim's job change and so depressed about leaving our home here that I couldn't help it. Fever went up to 99.6 that night, joints ached! I iced them, went to bed early, but couldn't sleep well.

Monday, August 3

Fever still at 99.6 at 11 A.M. Joints still hurt terribly. Bright red rash appeared on my neck and shoulders. I called my doctor, who prescribed more anti-inflammatory. Went to pharmacy, took meds, then went to bed.

Tuesday, August 4

Rash is worse! And now my joints are so sore I can hardly walk. I called my doctor again, and this time she said to come in. She drew blood, said I probably triggered a flare, increased my prednisone, and told me to rest.

Wednesday, August 5

Well, the pain is better, but the prednisone has me so hyped up I'm exhausted! And Jim's supposed to find out about the transfer tomorrow, so I'm still worried about that. I really wouldn't want to move, but he has to work to keep our insurance.

Thursday, August 6

Well, it looks like Jim won't be transferred, but now we won't know for sure until tomorrow. I'm feeling a little better about it, but we can't celebrate until we're positive. My joint pain is much better, and I took a nap today. My temperature's down, too, to 99. Whew!

Friday, August 7

Praise the Lord! Jim won't be transferred! I didn't know how worried I was until he found out we don't have to move! My pain is much better, and my temperature was normal all day. I haven't heard about my blood work yet; I wonder if everything's okay?

Saturday, August 8

Heard from my doctor late yesterday and my blood work was okay. I'm feeling much better. Slept really well last night, felt more in control. I played with the dog inside while Jim cut the lawn. Those squishy, soft toys sure do come in handy!

Lupus Diary

Similar to a symptom log, a lupus diary tracks your daily ups and downs coping with the disease. It includes the tips and tricks you've learned to use to make your life easier, and it chronicles your journey with lupus from early in your diagnosis to the present. It is especially useful when you are feeling low and wonder if you've made any progress. A quick review of your earlier days will show that you have, indeed, come a long way!

Sample Lupus Diary and Entries

Sunday, September 16

I was pretty upset when I saw the rash on my forearm. It wasn't there in the morning, and it looked really bad. My hair's falling out enough as it is. I sure don't want anything else going wrong! I'm going to call my doctor in the morning.

Monday, September 17

I went in to see my doctor and he raised my prednisone. Worse, Jim wants to take a vacation this year to the islands, but I don't have any fun there anymore because I can't be in the sun. I can only read so long, and it takes no time to shop in those tiny stores. I wish he'd be okay with going someplace else, but he's so stubborn! And I'm still worried about the blood test results, plus this prednisone is making me sooo bitchy and hungry! I feel like eating a whole pizza and throwing the box at the dog.

Friday, September 21

Can it get any worse?! I feel so hyper that I'm ready to pull my hair out—if it hadn't already fallen out! My wig looks horrible. My fingernails are all broken. And Jim wouldn't let me get that pizza last night. He made a huge salad instead.

Wednesday, September 26

Urghhh! I was up at 3 A.M. I vacuumed the downstairs, watched one of those awful infomercials, and actually bought those dust rags! Then I read the newspaper. Again. But nothing registered. Prednisone is my enemy! And Jim mentioned vacations again today.

Thursday, September 27

I can't imagine going on vacation. I can't imagine going away for the weekend. I can't even imagine a time when I won't have to be on this high a dose of prednisone. My life is a mess. The dog won't play with me. Jim's working late. I don't even want those dust rags, but they're going to show up here any day now.

Friday, October 12

I get to decrease my prednisone today, and I feel a little better already. Jim said he doesn't have to work quite as late. The dog wagged his tail.

Tuesday, October 23

Decreased prednisone a third time. Feeling much more in control. Jim came home from work early and gave me a beautiful bouquet of flowers. He's really a good guy. And I can't wait for our vacation! We're going to Seattle!

Specialized Logs

Sometimes your doctor will want you to track a specific symptom or get regular readings of, for example, your blood pressure or temperature. In this case, modify the symptom log so that you have all your readings on one easy-to-read page. A food diary may help to figure out whether a dietary trigger for migraine headaches or abdominal pain is present. The benefits of exercise to lupus activity, fatigue, and depression are not readily apparent until a patient charts his or her symptoms along with the exercise routine.

Here is an example of a temperature log:

TEMPERATURE LOG—AUGUST 2001
In Degrees
(All readings taken between 4:00 and 4:30 P.M. unless otherwise noted)

	Sun	Mon	Tues	Wed	Thurs	Fri	Sat
WEEK ONE:				98.6	99	99.2	99.4
WEEK TWO:	99.4	99	98.6	98.6	98.6	99.1	99.2
WEEK THREE:	99.2	98.6	98.6	98.6	98.6	98.6	98.6
WEEK FOUR:	99	99	99.2	99.2	99	99	99.1

Preparing for an Office Visit— Physician's Perspective

In the days of managed care and decreased reimbursement for office visits from insurance companies, many physicians find that they are not able to spend as much time as they would like with their patients. Some preparation on the patient's and physician's parts would help to make the most productive use of their time.

Having a list of your current medications on a notecard is

very helpful to keep your rheumatologist updated about any new medications started by other physicians. It is also helpful to note the names of medications that were tried and stopped in the past due to lack of efficacy or side effects. Write down a list of questions to ask your doctor and select two or three of the most important ones for your visit.

If you have seen other doctors or had tests performed before the visit, call the office or hospital in advance to make sure that a preliminary report or note has been sent to your rheumatologist.

If a symptom appears to be unusual, call ahead to your doctor and discuss the symptom in advance of your visit so that he or she can give some thought to your unusual symptom before your visit. Wear comfortable clothing and avoid wearing makeup if appropriate to make examination of knee joints and rashes easier.

Bring in a blood pressure, headache, or other symptom log when indicated. Obtain a copy of your laboratory work and keep a file of your tests so that they may be shared among other doctors that you see. Let your doctor know if you have had trouble with blood draws in the past so that thinner needles can be used.

Collect a twenty-four-hour urine specimen for protein estimation in order to assess the severity of kidney disease, and bring it in advance of your appointment if possible so that the results are available at the time of your appointment.

At your office visit, if a medication is prescribed, make sure you ask how to take it, when it should work, and what side effects to monitor. Use your own personal method to monitor for benefits such as a numerical scale of intensity of symptoms, days missed from work, or ability to perform more activity. Report this to your physician when you return for your next visit.

If you plan to visit your physician with a family member who has a question about your illness, or if there is an unusual symptom, call your physician a few days in advance of your visit so that he or she may research or prepare for that visit.

Physicians can help their patients by supplying them with copies of their lab tests, printed booklets about their illness and medications, and newsletters that have information about cutting-edge research on their illness.

8

THE MEDICAL FACTOR:

How to Survive
a Hospital Stay

No lupus patient wants to be hospitalized, and many never will be. But there might come a time when hospitalization is necessary, and the experience can be frightening. The usual reasons for hospitalization in the first year for a lupus patient include a kidney biopsy, seizures, or persistent fever due to active lupus or infection. Being prepared in the event of a stay makes life easier, as does having a positive outlook on why you are there and what to expect.

You Are Not Alone

Many lupus patients fear going to the hospital because they believe that it is the last resort. However, sometimes the best way to get better during a serious flare is to spend a few days in the hospital, where you can receive more consistent, thorough treatment.

"I've been hospitalized sixty times," says Becky, who was diagnosed in 1970 at the age of thirty. "But I never thought I was going to die from my problems. The purpose of the hospital is to get better."

As Becky has found from her experience, there are a number of factors that go into making a hospital stay a success. First among them is a positive attitude, but having the right medical team, including an advocate, is essential, too.

Health-Care Vigilance

With today's health crisis, shortage of nurses, and managed-care complications, you have to maintain vigilance over your care outside as well as inside the hospital.

Becky says, "You have to stay motivated and keep your wits about you. If you can't, you have to have someone who is your advocate."

The Advocate

Although you might be lucid during much of your hospital stay, there could be times when you will be sedated or otherwise less than clearheaded. At those times, you will need someone with you who can make sure that you receive appropriate, timely care. "For example," says Becky, "you have to make sure you get the right meds at the right time. And if you get a generic, know why."

An advocate can work with the hospital staff in making sure you receive your medication at the right time, notify your doctor or other person of changes in your condition, or just keep you company during the lonely, long hours.

The advocate can be a family member, a close friend, or a "lupus buddy." Another option is to hire a health-care worker to specifically focus on your case. Some private nursing agencies provide nurse advocates. Your physician, hospital, or local chapter of the Arthritis Foundation can help you locate a professional advocate, if that is what you need. Costs vary according to location, how many hours you need that person to be present, and what kind of credentials you require the advocate to have.

Whomever you choose, make sure the person is knowledgeable enough about what you would prefer in the way of care. Select someone who has a good sense of humor and is positive about your ability to get better. He or she should be coolheaded and able to make decisions calmly and logically. Also, choose someone who is willing to let you take charge when you can. You need to keep control of your health care as much as possible in order to maintain your interest and energy in getting better.

Family and Friends

Designate one close friend or family member as someone who can contact others and give them updates on your health. This will save you from having to repeat yourself, and will allay your loved ones' fears about your condition. It will also let them know when you can receive visitors and telephone calls, avoiding interruptions during your treatment or rest periods.

If you are in the hospital for more than a few days, chances are the stream of visitors and gifts might taper off. Don't be alarmed or think that people don't care about you anymore. Understand that their lives are full, too, and expect that you will pick up on your relationships when you are released.

Roommates and Other Strangers

Unless you are fortunate enough or wealthy enough to afford a private room, you will probably have to share your room with at least one other patient. That person might become a source of solace and company for you, or he or she might drive you crazy with complaining, visitors, noise, or other distractions.

If you are greatly bothered by your roommate, try to get your bed moved to another room. However, as crowded as hospitals are these days, this might not be possible. Express your need for rest, quiet, or privacy with the nurses on call and ask for their help in troubleshooting with your roommate. Above all, throughout your stay, be as pleasant as possible with your roommate; he or she is hurting, too.

Don't Just Lie There!

"I'm the worst patient to be put into the hospital," says Becky. "My first question is always, 'When am I getting out?' "

Indeed, from the moment you are admitted, your focus should be on getting better. Here are certain things you can do to make sure this happens:

- Know exactly why you are in the hospital and what your doctor or doctors prescribe as your treatment.
- Follow your doctor's orders and speak up about any side effects, changes in your symptoms, or discomfort.
- Insist on attention when you need it and respect the busy schedule of the nurses when you do not.
- Keep your mind active by reading, working puzzles, doing handiwork, or playing games with others.
- Welcome visits or phone calls from friends or family, but let them know when you need your quiet and rest.
- Pray and meditate; leave your worries about home and

family outside the walls of the hospital and dwell on the positive aspects of getting better.

- Contact the hospital's chaplain, rabbi, or priest and speak with him or her on a regular basis.
- You or the advocate should keep track of your dosages, making sure that you receive the proper medication at the assigned time and that all information is recorded accurately on your chart. If there are any changes, discuss them with the nurse on duty and your doctor.

Being patient is important, too, as is understanding that you are a consumer being provided with a service.

"You can fire and hire and deal with your doctors as much as you want," says LaTanya, a registered nurse and lupus patient. "Being in the hospital can be traumatic for anybody, but you have to maintain your total control."

While you are in the hospital, you will be treated and seen by a number of health-care professionals. Be aware that each will have his or her own style of treating you. However, if you experience unusual or severe pain during any procedure do not hesitate to speak up about it.

If you feel you are being treated unprofessionally, or experience any lapses in care or mistakes, report the experience to the supervisor. But do not be overly critical of things beyond anyone's control; hospitals are not hotels, nor is the experience meant to approximate that of a spa or resort.

Paperwork

One of the things people complain about most is the volume of paperwork accompanying a hospital stay. Forms have to be filled out before admittance, during your stay, and afterward. You have to keep close track of your insurance forms, too, and make sure that all charges are accurate and that they are settled properly.

Preparing for the onslaught of paperwork is key to making sure it is not overwhelming. Here are some tips:

- If possible, preregister with the hospital before you arrive. This includes getting a patient number and giving the hospital your insurance information, emergency contact numbers, and pertinent medical information. Ask if you can fill out paperwork prior to arriving. Keep a copy for your files.

- Ask your insurance company about coverage for the services you will receive in the hospital. Get the name of the person you speak with, and note the time and date of your call.
- Update your power of attorney, health-care directive, or other personal paperwork designating whom you want to make decisions for you in case you are incapacitated. Carry a copy of the necessary forms with you to the hospital. (If you don't, the hospital might want you to fill out its own forms when you arrive.)
- Carry two copies of a list of your current medications, your health history, and contact telephone numbers with you. Give one copy to your advocate and keep the other one, providing it to the hospital if asked.
- As best you can, keep track of the procedures and services you receive at the hospital. Match them up with what is charged on your bill or the Explanation of Benefits (EOB) that you receive from your insurance company. You may want to question charges for services that you think you did not receive.
- Obtain a Release of Information form from the hospital when you leave. About two weeks later, fax it to the hospital so that you can get important documents such as a discharge summary, test results, and procedure notes for your records.

Attitude

The right attitude can help you heal faster and speed up your release from the hospital. This means that you should try to avoid unnecessary complaining and follow all your doctor's orders. Keeping your sense of humor will fill the long hours you spend in bed, as will visiting with friends and family. And be sure to maintain contact with your inner peace; as hard as it might be to find quiet in the hospital, such activity will help you keep your emotional stamina at a high level and speed your release.

When You Get Out

Before you are released from the hospital, ask for a detailed list of all medications and activities you are supposed to (or not supposed to) take or engage in. Get a sense of the length of time you will need for a full recovery, and make any follow-up appointments necessary.

Expect a dip in your energy level in the days following your release, even if you are extremely eager to get out of the hospital. Remember that you have not been moving about as you are used to doing, and it will take some time to get your strength back to where it was before you were hospitalized. Make sure that you walk in the corridor of the hospital at least two to three times a day for at least ten minutes, if permitted to do so, in order to maintain muscle tone and endurance.

Do not be ashamed or embarrassed to rely on loved ones to help you make the transition from the hospital to the home. Appreciate their assistance and accept it as a wonderful gift that will help speed your recovery. Use your stay in the hospital as a way to better appreciate the world around you, the things you can do, and the loving people in your life.

Reasons for Hospitalization in a Lupus Patient

Lupus patients may be hospitalized when they present with seizures, strokes, or confusion due to brain involvement. Another common reason for admission is for persistent fever in spite of using antibiotics as an outpatient. Tests to rule out a hidden infection may be necessary in the hospital until aggressive treatment is directed at active lupus.

The first year after being diagnosed may be particularly stormy in the case of lupus patients with organ involvement. Patients with nerve, liver, or kidney involvement will often need to be admitted to the hospital for a biopsy, a procedure where a sample of tissue is obtained to establish the diagnosis and grade the severity of involvement.

A kidney biopsy helps to classify the severity of kidney disease and determine the right course of treatment. Usually, you will need to prepare for a kidney biopsy at home by checking your clotting time and stopping all medications that prevent the clotting of blood up to one week prior to the procedure.

A kidney biopsy is usually done in the prone position under local anesthesia so that the patient is conscious and can take a deep breath and hold it when the biopsy is performed. Mild sedatives may be used if a patient is very anxious.

In the proper hands, biopsies are safe, and the pain during and after the procedure can be managed with appropriate pain medications. Do not be afraid to ask your rheumatologist about the qualifications of the surgeon performing the procedure. You want a doctor who has performed several of these procedures in the past and is active in this field currently. Find out the adverse events that might occur with the procedure and how one can minimize them. For instance, if you stop taking aspirin and anti-inflammatory medication, you might help to decrease the risk of bleeding. Reducing the dose of prednisone and chemotherapy medicines helps to avoid infections. Also, try to time your procedure in the early morning, when your treatment team is alert and at their best.

9

The Financial Factor

Lupus can be an extremely expensive illness, especially because it is so unpredictable. Financial planning can be difficult as you experience unforeseen costs associated with medicines, doctor visits, and hospitalizations. Also, the things you need to do to adapt your life to lupus can be expensive; changing your home, your wardrobe, and your activities can bring about extra expenses and put a dent in your savings plan or discretionary income.

There are some ways that you can prepare yourself and your family for the ups and downs of a life with lupus. These include making sure you have adequate insurance and are prepared to meet deductible and copay expenses, becoming more "discount minded" when it comes to making purchases, and being sure to keep your inner spirit peaceful so that money matters do not cause you significant stress. But above all else it is important to regularly assess your financial situation and stick to a budget.

How Lupus Will Affect Your Budget

Obviously, your immediate expenses are those that command your most pressing attention. How you handle them will have an impact on your ability to withstand future, unpredictable costs. Budgeting is extremely important to make sure that you are able to meet your current needs; however, thinking about your present expenses with an eye toward your future needs as a lupus patient will help you enormously.

Insurance

You should consider your insurance expense as part of your necessary, current budget. Health, disability, automobile, and homeowner's (or renter's) insurance are all included in this category. All can help you weather catastrophic occurrences such as automobile accidents; fire, flood, or earthquake damage; or sudden hospitalization. Health insurance can also defray some of the cost of routine health care, including prescriptions, laboratory expenses, outpatient tests, and doctor visits.

Besides the effect on your bank statement and your standing as a good citizen, having insurance coverage can give you tremendous peace of mind when you consider all the what-ifs that life can bring. Knowing, for example, that you are covered if you need to be hospitalized enhances your peace of mind and thus can help speed your recovery. Health insurance coverage can also make you more inclined to seek medical advice when you develop non-life-threatening, but still discomforting, symptoms.

Shopping for the proper insurance can be a daunting, time-consuming task. In some areas, insurance brokers can give you more options than if you'd done the investigating yourself. Also, a broker can save you time that you would rather spend on your health or other activities.

Even if you rely on a broker to come up with options, you need to weigh each of them carefully, taking into account your current health, other needs, and financial status. Consider the ramifications of paying for a lower premium by opting for a higher deductible (do you have the deductible amount saved up already?), and carefully weigh all the types and levels of coverage against what your health condition needs are.

There are certain pitfalls to watch out for, too. It might be tempting to pay a very low premium to a not-very-well-known insurance company, but sometimes trouble can follow if the company suddenly disappears or goes into bankruptcy. You are better off selecting a company that comes highly recommended, is registered in your state (check with your state's insurance commissioner), and has a long track record of providing the coverage you are looking for.

When you are looking for health insurance after you have been diagnosed, your lupus might be considered a preexisting condition.

Sometimes this will make you ineligible for coverage, or you will have to wait for a period of time before lupus-related expenses are covered. Be patient, persistent, and truthful in your insurance search. Sometimes you will have to apply for more than one policy before you obtain coverage.

Once you have found the right insurance coverage, fit your payments into your monthly budget. Take advantage of having your premiums automatically withdrawn from your checking or savings account so that your payment status is current even if you are too ill or forget to write the premium check. Make sure that you are prepared to pay the deductible on your policy, and notify your physicians of your new insurance, billing address, and the insurance company's contact telephone number.

Why Are Lupus Drugs So Expensive?

New therapies for lupus are often gleaned from the field of transplantation or cancer therapy. These medications are usually developed for other illnesses at a very high research-and-development cost and are later applied to the treatment of lupus at the same price as treating cancer or transplant patients. The treatment of cancer is usually for a defined period of time, whereas lupus is a chronic illness requiring lifelong treatment. All new drugs are patent-protected for about seven years so that no competitors can force the price down. New "smart medicines" for lupus that target lupus-specific molecules are in development, but are likely to be expensive.

Medical Expenses

Other expenses that you can count on regularly are those associated with the treatment of your disease. These include doctor visits, medical supplies, and medication, all of which can become very costly.

If you have good insurance coverage, much of your cash outlay will be softened. However, you will still probably have deductibles,

The Cost of Treating Lupus

Effective treatment for lupus can be expensive, since lupus is a chronic illness. Costs for treatment can be divided into direct costs and indirect costs. Direct costs include the cost of doctor visits, prescription medications and aids, hospitalization costs, and the costs of procedures such as blood tests and X rays. Indirect costs of lupus include loss of work and changes in the home environment made necessary because of the illness.

Direct costs for a lupus patient with no major organ involvement range from $2,000 to $5,000 a year, of which half the costs can be attributed to doctor visits and necessary lab tests and procedures. Major organ involvement can increase the direct costs by $12,000 to $25,000 per year due to the need for more expensive treatments and the occasional need for hospitalization. Good health insurance policies may cover up to 80 percent of most direct costs, but copayments, deductibles, and treatments that are not covered can quickly add up to a sizable sum.

Indirect costs are not often readily apparent, yet these may often be more than the direct costs of treating lupus. Loss of workdays or inability to work is usually the biggest indirect cost to the individual, his or her family, and to society. Because lupus is a disease with debilitating fatigue and pain, it can lead to unpredictable sick days requiring doctor visits or rest at home. Other indirect costs include changing the home environment and one's wardrobe to be more "lupus friendly."

copayments, and out-of-pocket expenses not covered by insurance. Some of these include:

- Annual eye exams if you are taking Plaquenil
- Calcium in tablet form and supplemental vitamins
- Nonprescription nonsteroidal anti-inflammatories
- Regular dental exams (unless you have insurance coverage for this)

- Moisturizing products for eye, mouth, or vaginal dryness if you have Sjögren's syndrome
- Heating pads, hot and cold packs, and ointment for sore and stiff muscles and joints
- In-home medical care, extending to housekeeping and other errands if you are unable to do these yourself
- In-home medical therapeutic devices such as paraffin baths for sore hands and feet
- Reading material about your disease
- Memberships in foundations and organizations related to lupus, Sjögren's syndrome, etc.

If you set aside a certain amount of money each month, you will be able to defray some of the sting of having these expenses suddenly overwhelm you.

Planning for the Future

"How can I plan for the future when lupus is so unpredictable?" laments one lupus patient.

"Just when you think one problem is solved, another one crops up," says another.

"Living with lupus is like living with a terrorist. You never know when it's going to strike," says yet another.

True, lupus is completely, utterly bewildering, especially to someone uneasy with or unused to constant change. But that is no reason to give up making plans for the future. Certainly it is no reason to stop funding retirement savings accounts, looking forward to your children's education, or dreaming about the vacation you've always wanted to take.

Savings

Fewer people die from lupus than ever before. In fact, most lupus patients can look forward to a normal life span, albeit with a chronic disease in the picture. What does this mean to your finances?

First and foremost, it means you should not stop trying to save for future expenses. However, you may have to pare back the amount that you set aside in tax-deferred retirement savings accounts, such as IRAs or 401(k)s. With lupus, unexpected expenditures are chronic, so it's important to stay as liquid as possible.

Withdrawing funds from tax-deferred accounts can be difficult and will cost you. However, you should take advantage of your employer's 401(k) plans or other savings instruments as much as you can afford to.

TIP: Set Up More than One Savings Account

You may feel guilty about withdrawing money from savings to do something nice for yourself. Saving for other things, such as vacations and major expenses, is all right, too. You should not feel as though your life is over because of lupus! Setting up a separate medical expense savings account will help you provide for times when your health needs significant attention.

Retraining and Other Professional Education

As you assess your work situation, you might discover the need to modify your current job or prepare for another career. Such a transition takes careful planning, even for a "healthy" person. You will need a savings plan for future tuition and expenses, and a provision in your current budget so that you will be able to afford the financial expenditure of such a move. You might need to plan for it to take longer than the average time to complete a particular program, especially if you have a very active disease. This, too, can lead to extra expenses, especially if you end up repeating a course. And if you need help doing your work (for example, you need to employ a note taker because you cannot write quickly enough during class lectures), that, too, will add to your education expenses.

Disability Insurance

There could come a time when you will be unable to work at all. You will still need some form of income to pay for your expenses. Disability insurance policies are made for just that purpose, and it is a good idea for every adult to carry this coverage. However, if you did not have a private disability plan before you were diagnosed with lupus, it is unlikely that you will be able to get such coverage once you have been diagnosed.

Certain states offer short-term disability coverage, which is usually applied for by your physician. There is a waiting period before benefits begin, and the duration of coverage is generally no more than a year. Although the amount of money you may receive is usually not significant, it can help defray some of your medical expenses and help ease your financial worries.

Social Security Disability

If you expect to be disabled for a longer period of time than that covered by a state short-term disability policy, consider filing for Social Security Disability. If your claim is accepted, you could be paid a monthly sum based upon your past earnings from a specific period of time, and continue receiving benefits until you are eligible for regular Social Security at the age of sixty-five, or when determined by law.

To begin the process of filing a claim for receiving Social Security Disability benefits, call your local Social Security office, which will send you forms to complete, as well as schedule you for a telephone interview.

The information you give to Social Security will be added to medical records obtained from your physicians in order to complete your application file. It is essential that you provide complete and truthful details regarding your condition and the effect that it has on your ability to perform life- and work-related tasks. Also, it is important that your doctors provide notes and lab reports that support their diagnoses and evaluation. Because physicians and their staffs are inundated with forms and reports, you should follow up with each of your doctors to make sure they have filed their information with Social Security within the guidelines and deadlines set forth in the application protocol.

After you participate in the telephone interview and complete and return the application forms, your file will be reviewed and a decision will be rendered. Few of the initial requests for Social Security Disability coverage are approved in the first round. If you are rejected, you have the opportunity to appeal the decision. Be mindful of the time frame for returning the appeals forms and follow it carefully, as failure to do so could put your application back at square one.

Many people have found that having an attorney at the appeals level is helpful for them. Indeed, having an advocate can take much of the stress off of you as you continue in the application and appeals process. Also, disability law is constantly changing, and an attorney can keep you in compliance with the latest changes in the regulations.

Your local Lupus Foundation chapter, the Arthritis Foundation, or the State Bar Association can give you a list of attorneys who practice disability law. Such lawyers generally work on contingency, meaning they do not get paid unless you are granted and paid disability benefits.

In many cases, having Social Security Disability benefits also entitles you to health coverage under Medicare. Again, there is a waiting period for this. But for someone with no other options, such coverage can, literally, be a lifesaver.

Taxes and Other Concerns

When you have a chronic illness, you need to pay particular attention to the implication of medical expenses on your overall tax picture. Because tax laws are constantly changing, the best expert for questions about the current tax requirements and provisions, including what is deductible and what isn't, is a certified public accountant. Here is how you can best be prepared for your consultation with a CPA:

- Keep a log of all doctor visits you made during the past year, including the number of miles you drove to and from and any parking costs. If you did not drive, but took a taxi or other form of transportation, note this instead and include the cost of such travel.
- Save all receipts, even if you think the expenses are inconsequential; everything adds up to the full picture of how much you spent for your medical condition, and even if some of it is not tax deductible, it will ultimately help you plan for future expenses.
- Record how much you pay for medical insurance premiums, as well as how much the insurance company reimburses for expenses versus how much you pay out of your own pocket. Note and investigate all discrepancies between what the insurance company was billed and what services you actually received.
- Don't forget expenses such as eye exams, glasses and contact lenses, and dentist visits in your itemization.

When you have determined how much you spent on medical services, supplies, and medications, draw at least an estimation of how much you are likely to spend in the coming year and figure that amount into your annual budget. This way you are less likely to have surprises when those expenses come up again.

It is always best to be prepared for the inevitable, so track your medical expenses and receipts continuously throughout the year. Not having to do a lot of reconstruction and last-minute searching for receipts and figures will relieve you of a lot of stress and speed up the process of getting a refund, if you are due one.

Estate Planning

More lupus patients than ever before can look forward to a nearly normal life span. So in many ways, planning for what happens to your estate after your death is no different now than it was before you had lupus. It is prudent to have a will that outlines all the provisions you wish to make for your assets, and provides for guardianship for any minor children you might have.

In addition to the usual provisions regarding disbursement of your assets, you should also have a living power of attorney, which will designate someone to look after your assets and your physical care should you be unable to do so yourself. In extreme circumstances, a special-needs trust might be appropriate, as well. Your family attorney and certified public accountant can help you determine what is advisable in your particular case.

Another question that often arises regarding end-of-life decisions is whether lupus patients can be organ and tissue donors. In most cases, unfortunately, the answer is no. Because of the medications and disease process specific to most lupus patients, donating tissues and/or organs is not advisable after the patient's demise. Likewise, it is not advisable for a lupus patient to consider donating blood, a kidney, bone marrow, or other body parts during his or her lifetime.

Defraying Expenses

With the added burden of medical bills and lifestyle adaptations, most lupus patients experience "disease sticker shock." Creative planning and research will yield many ways to help you survive the high cost of lupus.

Working as a Family to Cut Back Financially

If you stop working because of your lupus, or if you take a less stressful and thus less lucrative job, you will feel a financial pinch. It could be difficult to pare back your expenses to fit in with your new salary.

If your family depends upon your salary to sustain it, you should explain to everyone the reasons why you are cutting back on working. Let them know that you don't love them any less; rather, you want to be present for them, and the best way to do that is for you to have less stress on your health.

Ask your family members, children included, to list the things that they find are most important to them, the must-haves. Work with your children to understand that the most important things are really not frills, but basics such as food, clothing, lodging. Make up substitutes for more expensive activities or things. Alternatives might include:

- Having family "cook at home" nights instead of eating out
- Renting movies instead of going to the theater
- Decreasing the number of television sets in the household to one and watching programs as a family—and talking about them
- Making weekly outings to the museums, libraries, and parks in the area
- Playing board games at home—and just being together as a family

"People who need a lot of possessions have a harder time," says Penny. "As long as I can pay for my food, rent, and clothes, I'll be okay."

Health Insurance

Group plans, available through your employer, union, or trade association or guild, are usually the least expensive in terms of premiums. If you do not have access to any of these options and are on Social Security Disability (SSD), you might qualify for Medicare coverage. Your state might also have provisions for supplemental coverage for those patients on disability who have low incomes.

Getting your own health insurance through a major insurance company can be extremely costly or impossible due to your medical condition. Some states have begun to offer "high-risk" policies to people whose medical histories preclude them from getting their own private coverage. Check into this possibility by contacting your state insurance commissioner.

Medication

Some pharmaceutical companies sponsor programs that will provide certain medications to people who need them but cannot otherwise afford them. If you find yourself in dire straits, contact the pharmaceutical company that makes the drug you need and ask about their "patient assistance program" (also known as the "indigent patient assistance program").

New medications can be particularly expensive. Sometimes pharmaceutical companies or doctors' offices will participate in clinical trials for cutting-edge treatments. If you fit the criteria for a study, you could receive medication at no cost. Sometimes participants are paid, too! If you are interested in taking part in a trial, speak with your doctor and review the notices in publications put out by the Arthritis Foundation and the Lupus Foundation to find out what the new trials are and who to contact to find out more information about them.

To defray the cost of medicines, sometimes you might be tempted to switch from a brand to a generic. Check with your doctor before making such a move; the dollars you think you will save might not be worth it. If your insurance company will not pay for brand drugs, still make sure, through your doctor, that your treatment will not be compromised. And if your pharmacist suddenly switches you from brand to generic, insist that he or she refill your prescription to what it was before; consistency is very important.

Medical Services

If you have inadequate health insurance coverage, do not go without medical care because of it! Discuss your situation with your doctor and see if you can work out a satisfactory and doable payment schedule. If he or she is not willing to work with you, contact your local Arthritis Foundation or Lupus Foundation chapter for referrals to physicians who might be of more assistance.

Also, investigate the clinics and hospitals in your area to see if one of them might provide you with care, if only on an interim basis. Above all, do not turn to unorthodox treatments, unlicensed "professionals," or other backroom alternatives. The consequences could be harsh, even deadly.

Services

Do you need someone to do your gardening because you can no longer spend time in the sun? Does your Raynaud's make it impossible for you to shovel your driveway?

Ask a neighbor to help you, and do something for him or her in return. Barter arrangements might have tax implications (check with your accountant); however, they can be indispensable in many situations.

Coupons, Clubs, and Other Sources of Savings

If you shop at a store regularly, ask if they have a frequent buyers' club, or something similar. Sometimes the nominal membership fee is worth the amount of savings you can count up during the course of the year. Watch the newspaper and magazines for discounts, too, in the form of short-term sales and coupons.

Once again, the Internet can be a place to find savings. There are even Web sites that offer discount coupons redeemable at local grocery stores. A brief time browsing through cyberspace can save you a bundle!

Buying bulk items with your friends is another way to save. One lupus support group ordered multiple copies of publications regarding setting up a health-care directive. The price per piece went down the more copies they ordered, so everyone benefited from the purchase.

Where to Get Help

The burden of paying for a chronic disease can become overwhelmingly stressful whether you are on your own or married and with a family. Before you consider drastic measures, such as filing for bankruptcy, talk to your doctor or therapist to get suggestions and guidance about what else you can do. A certified public accountant can review your tax status to see if there are areas where you can gain savings and ease your burden. Also, consider getting in touch with your community's Consumer Credit Counseling Service. Such a service is usually free and can be very helpful, particularly if you are deeply in debt.

In the midst of your financial challenges, continue to work on your inner self. Pray and meditate, and use visualization to "see" where you would like your life to go. If you support yourself internally, you will be better able to tackle your external troubles.

10

THE FINANCIAL FACTOR:

The Lupus Consumer

A lupus patient must often wear different eyes and ears when shopping for certain items, such as automobiles. This is because some purchases must be tailored to fit the patient's specific needs (such as ease of getting in and out of a car, tinting on the windows, etc.). Besides automobiles, there are many other items that should be analyzed appropriately before purchase. To do an accurate analysis, the lupus patient should use the following skills:

- **Objectivity:**
Some things that you want would be uncomfortable, harmful, or impractical for you to use. Make a list of all pros and cons before purchasing a big-ticket item, and look at the need for certain features or add-ons, not just the desirability of them.
- **Creativity:**
Consider out-of-the-box sources for information about products that are hard for you to find. For example, if you are looking for comfortable shoes, consult with people who spend a lot of time on their feet (such as nurses or waitresses) to learn what they do to combat foot fatigue, as well as where they find their shoes.
- **Financial Sense:**
Even if you are looking for very unusual or expensive items, there could be hidden discounts and other cost perks if you

look hard enough for them. For example, some clubs and alumni associations offer discount programs for a variety of companies and services. Special-needs organizations can also be helpful, especially if you are looking for medical devices or other health-related tools or supplies. If you are considering going back to school, there are regular scholarships available, as well as those offered specifically to those people with disabilities. It might take some digging to find these sources of savings, but your extra work could pay off greatly in the end.

• **Assertiveness:**
Lupus can be a very expensive disease, even if you take all precautions to pare down your expenses. You need to be sure that you get your money's worth at all times—in the doctor's office, at home, on the road, and everywhere in between.

• **Patience:**
This is a worthwhile skill to use when seeking a specific item for a specific use. Carefully consult all your resources (personal references, Internet searches, telephone book, trade associations, club and organization lists, newspaper advertisements) before you settle upon something that isn't exactly what you want or need.

Big-ticket Items

There are some purchases that are not made very often in your lifetime, but when they are, they require extra vigilance and thoughtfulness, especially for the lupus patient.

Automobiles
Consider the following when looking for a new car:

• **Comfort and Ease of Handling**
Automatic transmission will alleviate much of the wear and tear to your hands and legs that is caused by shifting gears, and automatic brakes will help foot and leg pain to ease up, too. A car with a good steering system and excellent visibility will make it easier for the lupus patient to maneuver, thus cutting down on driving stress and unnecessary movement.

• **Accessibility**
The height of the seats makes a huge difference in how easy

or painful it is to get in and out of a car. For example, a sports car might look stylish, but can be terribly painful to get in and out of if you have severe joint involvement. Controls that are within easy reach will contribute to your comfort, as well as safety.

• Sun Protection

Window tinting can help the lupus patient avoid the harmful rays of the sun and cut down on glare that could aggravate sensitive eyes. On many new cars, such tinting is standard issue and gives very strong protection against the sun's rays. However, on older models, most windows are either tinted very little or not at all.

• Reliability

If the car breaks down, you might find yourself stuck on a hot road, waiting for the tow truck. Besides bringing on extra stress, this could also expose you to the sun's harmful rays and noxious fumes from other passing vehicles.

• Climate Control

A good ventilation system is very important, as is a good air-conditioning and heating system that will filter out harmful particles while keeping you and your heat-sensitive lupus comfortable.

• Affordability

Make sure that financing can be worked out so that you are not using all your savings on the car and have nothing left for your health care or other purchases, including regular, essential car maintenance. Assess how much the upkeep on your car will be, and make your purchase based on long-term, as well as immediate, cost considerations.

How to find a comfortable, reliable, safe, affordable car is not an easy question to answer, but there are sources that can point you in the right direction.

- Ask your friends and other lupus patients what kind of cars they drive. Perhaps one or more of them will let you take a test drive, and you can get a firsthand idea of the different options without having to do so with a pushy car dealer.
- Ask your insurance broker or agent if he or she has any ideas about good-quality cars (which ones tend to have the most problems, etc.).

Window Tinting

Before you invest in having your car's windows tinted, there are several things you should look into:

- The reliability of the process and company you are employing to apply the tinting.
- The legality of the extent of the tinting you want to apply—in some states, dark tinting, particularly on the windshield, is illegal, while in others you will need a permit or note from your doctor so that your tinting is legal. To verify the legal issues related to window tinting, contact your state's Department of Motor Vehicles. In the state of California, contact the California Highway Patrol.
- The safety of the tinting in relation to your line of visibility in the car.

- Consult with consumer publications on the Internet and at the newsstand.
- Calling towing services and asking what cars they have to pick up most might yield some interesting and useful answers.

Where You Live

Your home is where you will spend most of your time, so it is especially important that it be a refuge, a place of comfort, ease, and rest. Whether you are buying a house or renting an apartment, naturally you will want someplace that is affordable and in a good location, too. Here are some other things to consider:

- **Location in relation to medical care, including pharmacies and hospitals.** You might get sick during the day or in the middle of the night. Think of how easy it would be to get to the proper medical treatment at whatever hour you might need it.
- **Direction and number of windows, and availability of air-conditioning system.** Be aware that sun and heat expo-

sure do not occur only outdoors. Choose a home so that you will be protected inside and out.

• **Number and type of stairs in and around the house.** Find a floor plan that is easy to navigate on your good and bad days.

• **Ease of maintenance inside the house.** Vaulted ceilings, elaborate woodwork, and other lovely but difficult-to-clean places might look fantastic, but pose problems for you if you intend to clean them in the midst of a flare.

• **Need for frequent, numerous repairs, remodeling.** If you choose a house that needs a lot of work, consider the effect that dust, confusion, and noise will have on your health.

• **Accessibility of property vis-à-vis nearby neighbors, roads, emergency vehicles.** Consider your proximity to neighbors, who might lend a hand if you are incapacitated or if there is an emergency. Also, determine how close or how far away you want and need to be from family and others who will be involved in helping you, especially during the rough periods. Make sure the house is easily accessible, even in winter, in case emergency vehicles need to get through.

• **Quality of water, air, soil around home.** Find out if the quality of the water and soil is such that you do not have to worry about being exposed to noxious chemicals.

• **Children- and Parent-friendly.** If you have children, think about their activities and how easy it will be to accommodate them in terms of transportation and your own vigilance. Assess how far you are willing to drive them to school, after-school activities, and friends' houses.

Computers and Other Technological Items

A computer in the home, particularly one that is hooked up to the Internet, can be a great asset to you. Purchasing a system can be confusing, and because technology is always changing, it is difficult to pinpoint what the best system is, overall, for the lupus patient. However, there are some guidelines to consider, whether you are new to the computer market or are considering an upgrade to your present system:

• **The monitor.** The size of the monitor should be large enough to view comfortably. You should be able to adjust the color, brightness, and clarity of the image on the screen.

- **The keyboard.** There are many different configurations of keyboards on the market today. Test several varieties and consult with your occupational or hand therapist to find one that accommodates your needs.
- **The mouse.** Many styles, from palm-held to button, exist. Again, test several and rely on your occupational or hand therapist to select the right one for you.

Additional devices and suggestions for making computer use easier are:

- Work with your occupational or hand therapist to devise a schedule for working on the computer, figuring in frequent breaks and, possibly, hand exercises to accommodate your health concerns.
- Use a wrist and hand brace on one or both hands to give yourself extra support when typing.
- Try out voice-recognition software, which can cut down on the number of keystrokes you make and ease the stress on your fingers and wrists.
- Set up your computer so that your back and arms are properly supported. Test several models of desk chairs to find one that is the right size and shape for you.
- Cut down on the glare that might come in from a window or from a lamp or light fixture.

Higher Education and Retraining

If you can still work but, because of your symptoms, must find another career or type of job, you will probably need to find a specific, specialized training program. Even if such education can be done at home, there can be a high cost associated with tuition, fees, and learning materials, not to mention the time and effort you will spend going through the program.

• Financial Assistance

Consult with scholarship books and Web sites that are geared toward financial aid for "healthy" people, as well as for those with disabilities. One such site, sponsored by the President's Committee on Employment for People with Disabilities (www.pcepd.gov), has a list of scholarships available, as well as other valuable information. Also, many local Arthritis

Foundation chapters offer scholarships, and the national office can provide you with even more information about them.

• **Study Assistance**

Contact the school or trade group responsible for the program you wish to enter and ask if they make any special accommodations for people with disabilities, including providing services that will make your study easier. Some universities will give disabled students voice-recognition software, offer access to note takers (people who sit in class with you and take notes), and provide transportation to and from classes. Usually, such help is free of charge to the student. Consider distance learning. Many institutions of higher learning offer coursework or degree programs over the Internet. Taking classes on-line gives you more flexibility if you're homebound for a time.

• **Lifestyle Assistance**

If you are totally disabled, you still might want to explore taking a class or entering a program that will be interesting for you, give you a better sense of yourself, and keep your hand in things outside your immediate circle. Scholarships and grants might also apply in this case—be sure to ask and investigate them. You never know until you try!

The "Little" Things

Today more than ever manufacturers are becoming aware of the vast population that is aging and in need of some help with basic devices and tools, such as cooking utensils. So it is easier to locate items that can make your life easier and less painful. However, be aware that some of those items are accompanied by high costs; careful and creative shopping can reveal similar items at significant savings.

Household Items

If you have lupus, you will spend a lot of time at home. As you find out about how lupus affects you, assess your home based on your needs and preferences.

• Invest in tools and appliances that will make your life easier and safer.

- Dispose of extraneous items that you will probably never use (old appliances, for example). Donate some of them to charitable organizations.
- Shop in catalogs, on the Internet, and through discount kitchen-supply stores to find the best item for the best price. Go to a hands-on store so that you can test items (hold them, practice lifting them, know exactly how they function) before purchasing them.

Clothing

Take your time finding clothing that fits, gives you the proper sun coverage, and appeals to your sense of style. Locate items at thrift shops, hospital boutiques, and discount stores. Be realistic about your medical condition and needs so that you will not waste money and thus not have the funds to buy clothes that *are* practical and attractive.

Other clothing tips to keep in mind are:

• Foundations
Besides your outer garments, give thought and attention to what you wear underneath them. Sometimes knowing you are wearing attractive undergarments can give you an added boost of confidence, too!

• Old Clothes
Save your old clothes for a time, in case your weight goes up or down.

• Hats
Have fun with hats! If you are a woman, try a man's hat sometime and see how stylish it looks! Dress up your old hats with pins, scarves, and other decorations to give them a new, updated look.

• Clothing Care
Save money by taking proper care of your clothes so that you can enjoy them longer. Invest in a good stain remover. Utilize services such as cobblers, who can repair shoes, handbags, and luggage, so that you can refresh your wardrobe and get more longevity out of favorite items.

• Share
Organize a fashion show for your lupus support group, either by inviting local vendors to show you what they have to offer or by bringing in favorites of your own. You can learn from one another's fashion experiences, find new sources of affordable clothing, and have a great deal of fun besides.

Luxury Items

Jewelry and other items might seem like luxuries, but they can brighten your day if you are feeling particularly low or unattractive. And they need not be expensive, either!

- Explore flea markets and garage sales early in the day, to avoid the sun and beat the crowds.
- Shop in thrift stores.
- Make your own styles out of materials you can purchase at hobby and craft stores.
- Gather some of your lupus friends together and practice making jewelry and other adornments together, perhaps selling some of them to make money to support the activities of your support group or lupus community.

TIP: Develop "Diplomatic Assertiveness"

When it comes to speaking up about the services and goods that you purchase, try to develop a greater sense of urgency that what you spend your money on must be worth the cost *and* helpful to your health. Learn to overcome any fear of confrontation. This does not mean that you rant and rave, stomp your foot, or threaten bodily harm. But it does mean that you state your needs calmly and, if the service or good that you are offered does not meet your needs, reject it, ask for a refund, and assert your position as the person spending the money.

When you buy clothing, for example, make sure that it is worth the cost in terms of fit, functionality, and fashion. If the garment falls apart or otherwise does not live up to its promise, follow the store's instructions about returns and take it back. If you do not get immediate satisfaction, ask—calmly—to speak with a supervisor who is authorized to give you the answer you need and deserve.

Diplomatic assertiveness takes time to develop, but it is worthwhile for several reasons. First, you learn to overcome any fear of confrontation. Second, it helps you get the services and goods that you need and pay for. Third, it gives you a greater sense of control; you are less of a victim if you can articulate and receive what you need. Fourth, it will relieve you of the stress of being dissatisfied, helpless, and victimized—all emotions that work against your struggle to maintain your inner peace while living with lupus.

Begin practicing diplomatic assertiveness in small ways to build confidence. Consider situations where you might stand up for yourself as an opportunity to practice. If you are unsure whether a situation calls for action on your part, talk it over with friends or your lupus support group.

11

THE PRODUCTIVITY FACTOR:

Lupus and the Workplace

As you know, lupus flares can preclude you from working or doing other things that make you feel like a productive member of society. This can, in turn, rob you of your self-worth and make you doubt your place in the world around you. You could become depressed, and your treatment could suffer, making it even more difficult to come out of a flare and reengage in life activities.

To Make the Impractical Work

There is no getting around it: Lupus is a very disruptive disease. Sometimes it might seem as though your whole life revolves around doctor visits, taking medication, coping with side effects, and canceling plans because you are too tired or too sick.

With lupus in your life, you have to take extra care that you will be able to keep up with your new goals and priorities, especially your health. This takes a lot of time, and several attempts, before you will feel comfortable.

And the first thing you should learn is to say no.

> ## TIP: The Right of Refusal
>
> If you listen to your body and are realistic about what you hear, you know there are times when you should stay home instead of going out, ask for help instead of doing something on your own, or request special accommodation rather than "grinning and bearing" a situation and suffering for it later.
>
> Remember that in all cases, even where family obligations are concerned, you have the right to say no. Even more than that, you have an obligation to your health to avoid putting yourself in harmful situations.

Communicating Your Priorities

Usually people will be reasonable if you explain that you have a medical condition that precludes you from doing something or taking on a certain responsibility. But they will not be reasonable, they will not understand, if you do not take the time to explain it to them.

This doesn't mean that you launch into a university-level explanation of lupus and its consequences, but it does mean that you give a simple, straightforward answer to their request, then stick by your decision. Sometimes providing additional information, such as a pamphlet from the Lupus Foundation, will help reinforce what you tell them. So will using a few well-thought-out analogies (such as explaining that joint pain feels like severe arthritis).

Sometimes constant communication is necessary. For example, some people will assume that you should be completely well in a few days, weeks, or months. They might not understand the nature of a chronic illness. Again, be patient but firm. You cannot expect people to understand if you do not explain.

Career Development and Goal Setting

One of the biggest questions facing lupus patients who are employed at the time of their diagnosis is, "What will happen to my career? Will I be able to work?"

In many cases, lupus patients will be able to work. In other cases, symptoms will preclude them from continuing in the same job or profession, but they might find fulfillment, and employment, elsewhere. Even for a patient who is told he or she cannot continue to work, having goals is still important to maintaining hope, health, and a good quality of life.

As you look at your situation and try to see into the future professionally, enlist the help of your doctor and fellow patients. Know what is harmful and what is helpful for you to do, and get suggestions from your friends, too.

If there is something you have always wanted to accomplish professionally, don't shelve that desire. Investigate what it will take to follow through, then map out a plan that will accommodate your health considerations while enabling you to see the possibility of achieving your goal. Keep this in mind, even when you feel too sick to see beyond your pain. Flares come and go; goals can be achieved in the times when you are feeling well enough to see your dreams become realities.

Some people who are diagnosed with lupus are not able to continue working. Their disease has progressed to the point where medical treatments and physical constraints preclude their being able to sustain their old jobs and careers.

Other people, however, are able to continue to work, or find that changing jobs or careers will help them maintain their sense of productivity while accommodating their lupus.

Deciding which way to go will take some thinking and talking— especially with your doctor and your spouse or loved ones.

Criteria for Making the Decision

Before you decide whether or not to continue working, you should take into consideration these things:

- ➤ Your doctor's opinion and recommendations
- ➤ Your current employer's willingness or ability to make accommodations for your lupus-related limitations
- ➤ Your need to sustain working at your current pace/occupation—the financial aspects of quitting or moving on
- ➤ The possibility of retraining, changing careers, or taking on a different occupation instead of leaving the workforce altogether

Your Doctor's Input

Not only does your doctor know your medical history, he or she also should know enough about how lupus affects patients to give you an idea of whether your current work situation will help or hurt your health. When you discuss a course of treatment for your lupus, have a detailed conversation with your physician about the following:

- Your current work-related duties and what you can and cannot do on the job
- The level of stress at your current job and the sources of that stress
- The potential you have for being flexible with your duties or hours
- Your needs (financial, personal, and familial) related to your employment

After having this discussion, ask your doctor what he or she thinks about your working. You might find that simple modifications will enable you to continue contributing in your present job. You might even find that no accommodations are necessary and that prudent care for your overall health will keep you working and productive.

However, you and your doctor might come to the conclusion that you need to cut back on your work duties, or stop working altogether. If that time comes, take a deep breath and lots of time to let it sink in. Going from working to not working is a financial, familial, and emotional shock. You will need patience and much positive thinking to adjust.

Telling Your Employer about Lupus

If you do not have a severe disease and do not need special accommodations in order to continue working, you might not even need to inform your employer that you have lupus. Most employers allow for a certain number of sick days, and if you do not feel well because of lupus, you should be able to avail yourself of the insurance, sick days, and consideration due every employee.

If you do have a severe disease, but your doctor has agreed you can continue to work within certain guidelines, you will probably have to tell your employer that you have lupus and, if directed by your doctor, request accommodation.

The Americans with Disabilities Act

Lupus is a condition that is covered under the Americans with Disabilities Act (ADA). According to the ADA, "all employers, including State and local government employers with 25 or more employees after July 26, 1992, and all employers, including State and local government employers with 15 or more employees after July 26, 1994," must comply with the ADA. They do not need to accommodate everything, however; the ADA specifies that they must give "reasonable accommodation" to employees with conditions falling under ADA protection. So if you request that you be allowed to work half days at full-time pay, you might not be accommodated. However, if you need an ergonomically better computer keyboard, your employer might be required to get one for you.

Information about the ADA and what it means to you is available in various places, including the United States government Web site: www.disability.gov.

Having the Discussion

Many employers have handbooks that outline the steps for reporting a disabling condition to the company, and many of them also have information relating to modifying work schedules and duties. The first place to look for guidance on how to approach your employer about what you need is the handbook and any other information your employer has on what the company provides. After you have read the handbook, make an appointment to speak with the appropriate person (supervisor, manager, etc.), and prepare for the meeting as you would for any work-related project.

It is best to approach your employer reasonably when you ask for accommodation. Provide him or her with information about lupus (many employers won't know what it is), and give your assurance that you want to be a contributing, productive member of your employer's team.

"I've always been extremely responsible and dedicated to my work," says Penny, age fifty-seven. "When I told my boss I have lupus, I explained that it wasn't something I wanted to discuss on a daily basis. I didn't want him to feel like he had to ask me, 'How are you feeling?' every day."

Ask for your employer's assistance in communicating your condition and any limitations to your coworkers, especially if you feel there will be a problem. Keep the lines of communication open between you and your employer; you do not need to give an office-visit-by-office-visit account of how you are faring, but you should be prepared to provide your employer with any information that he or she needs to verify your condition and work-related limitations.

Above all, be intent upon focusing on doing your job.

"I make my doctor appointments as conveniently as possible," says Penny. "And I don't want my boss to tell anyone else I have lupus. I don't want other people saying, 'Oh, poor baby.' I'm not looking for their sympathy. I want to focus on my job to the best of my ability."

Coworkers

You might be able to work without telling your coworkers about your lupus, and some lupus patients admit that this is best. However, if you need significant accommodation, you might need to tell those employees who work closely with you. And when you do, you might be surprised at their reactions.

Some of your coworkers might be fearful that you will shirk your duties and all the work will fall to them. They might resent your "special treatment" and take it out on you. They also might worry about their own health, or think that lupus is contagious.

Discuss your concerns with your supervisors, and provide them and your coworkers with enough information about lupus to alleviate their fears of contagion. Be open to suggestions that might ease the burden for your coworkers, as well as yourself. Try to put on your coworkers' shoes, just as you hope they will try to empathize with you. And again, stay focused on your work. Rely on your outside support system to handle your concerns about your symptoms and overall health.

Changing Jobs

If you leave your current job and transition into another line of work, you will, understandably, be nervous. This nervousness can cause stress, which can exacerbate your lupus. If you keep your mind on what is positive about your transition, you can lessen much of the stress and enjoy the change more.

Moving from a job full of responsibility and prestige (not to mention stress) can be a blow to your ego. But if you keep your focus on what is best for you, you will be able to weather it.

"Going from being a manager to being in a clerical position, like I had to do, could be a comedown, if that's what I got my esteem from," says Penny. "I try to remind myself that I can be me, that people can or cannot like me, but I'll still be okay."

One hopes you will choose a new career that will afford you less health aggravation and just as much if not more self-satisfaction as your old job. Take the transition slowly, keeping in mind that you also have a "job" when it comes to taking care of your health. And enjoy the freshness, the adventure of your change in direction. The more positive you are, the more benefits you will get from your new career.

Keep Your Doctor Up-to-Date

As you continue to work, include employment issues and duties on the job in the list of activities you provide for your doctor appointments. He or she will be able to see if there is a correlation between your lupus symptoms and work activities and might be able to make suggestions about modifications. Also, your doctor will be able to tell if working is, inevitably, too much for you to handle.

There might come a time when you will have to stop.

Leaving the Workplace Because of Disability

Before you were diagnosed with lupus, you may have thought you would not leave the workplace until you retired. However, unlike retiring or winning the lottery, leaving your job because of disability due to a chronic illness can be devastating. Instead of planning for a long stretch of time when you can do whatever you want, you will need to take on a new job—caring for your health. And that can be the most painful and difficult job you have ever had.

Leaving your job means that you will cease being in the company of coworkers, some of whom have become friends during the course of your tenure. If you have no children at home and your spouse works, or if you live alone, you will find long stretches of time when you are by yourself. This can stir up all your worries and preoccupations about your illness and contribute to a decline in your emotional stamina.

Disability Process

Employers, states, and the federal government have their own processes for applying for disability coverage and benefits. The amount of paperwork involved can be overwhelming, particularly if you are very ill. Also, you will sometimes need to go through one or more independent medical exams so that the agency or company through which you are applying can verify your condition. Such exams, added onto your regular medical checkups and treatment, can become very difficult to handle.

The better organized you are going into the application process, the better off you will be. If you are applying for Social Security Disability, you might consider hiring an attorney to help you through the process. Enlisting the services of a professional can take some of the burden and worry off of your shoulders—and that can help you cope so much better.

Financial

There are other financial considerations to leaving the workforce. You will need to find a way to pay for medical bills, keep up a savings plan, provide for your children (if you have any), and keep some extra money handy for being good to yourself. To be able to meet these needs, you will have to tackle your budget with new vigor, even if you don't have the energy to do so.

Being Unemployed

Not working also leaves a void in one of the areas you should pay close attention to even if you are very ill: your productivity. You are no longer subject to work-related projects, deadlines, and reviews. But you should still find something productive to occupy at least part of your time. Otherwise, you could fall into a deep depression driven by a lack of self-worth and self-esteem.

When you were employed, you had a structure and a schedule that helped keep order in your life. Having more of a structure enabled you to budget your time wisely. Once you are out of that structure, you might find your household "falling apart," and errands and chores might go undone. The television might seem mesmerizing, and the stack of magazines and catalogs alluring.

Now that you are not working, you will need to have a way to allocate your time so that you keep up with your responsibilities *and* your health care. Yes, you will need much time to rest. But keeping order in your house will help you feel better, more in control of your life.

Not as Bad as It Seems

Key to turning the lupus experience into a positive one is the realization that your productivity level and type might change, but it need not vanish. Perhaps you can no longer work full-time, or even part-time. Seek out ways of volunteering, where your schedule can be more flexible. Become involved with a support group and serve as a resource for other lupus patients. Reach out to the needy, the sick, or the lonely in your community. Helping others can be an excellent way of putting your own disease in perspective and giving you a deeper appreciation for the mobility and talents that you possess.

TIP: Think of Your Health as Your Job

Look upon the times when lupus keeps you housebound or bedridden as productive for your health. Taking care of yourself should be part of your job, and you should look upon it with the same seriousness and attention that you would give any other professional endeavor. Your salary is the degree to which you come out of the flare, and the perks are endless!

The Volunteer Alternative

The list of organizations and individuals who need assistance throughout the country is endless. In your own community, there are undoubtedly places and people who would welcome your skills and care. If you find that you cannot work a regular job, consider volunteer opportunities as a way to keep active, work with others, and contribute to doing good in a significant way.

Many nonprofit organizations use volunteers to form the backbone of their operations. Churches, synagogues, and community centers always need people to help with outreach and other services. The Lupus Foundation of America, the Arthritis Foundation, and other health-related groups are run mainly by volunteers and can even train interested people to lead support groups, exercise programs, and other more specialized activities.

As a volunteer, you can learn new skills, meet new people, and regain your sense of productivity while helping those less fortunate. You might find your experience leading to paying work, too; however, you should consider the benefits from volunteering as intrinsic to the experience itself. Take the pressure off of yourself to "get ahead," and enjoy your volunteer status instead.

Inner Strength

Throughout your day, as you grapple with the challenges of having lupus, make sure that you maintain touch with your inner self and cultivate your own core of peace.

Above all, know that your occupation does not define who you are, nor does your worth come from it. In fact, you are more important than a job, a paycheck, or a title. And the difference you can make in your life and others' goes far beyond any of those things.

12

THE PRODUCTIVITY FACTOR:

Lupus and the Home

As a lupus patient, sometimes it will seem to you that you spend all your time at your doctor's office, your "home away from home." Actually, much of your time will probably be spent at home. But, as with everything else, you may need to take a fresh look at your home. Does it support you, make your life a little easier as you reside with lupus? Or do you find where you are living more a hindrance than a help?

Productivity at Home

While home is a source of comfort, it is also a place that demands upkeep. The many chores and tasks our homes demand of us can sometimes become too much. However, there are changes you can make in your daily routine that can prove to be beneficial to you and your loved ones.

If your hands become so sore that cooking is a chore, perhaps your spouse can do it. You say he doesn't know how to cook? Suggest that one way he can help you with your lupus is by taking cooking classes. Let him know you'd be a willing "tester," even when the smells from the kitchen might make you wonder!

Do you usually do all your housekeeping—dusting, vacuuming, scrubbing floors—even when you're screaming with pain or bleary-eyed with fatigue? Perhaps you can invest in a cleaning service even once a month that will take care of the heavier chores for you. Although you might not think you can afford it, you might be able to find low-cost help through your local hospital or church. There is no defeat in admitting you need help in this area. You'd be surprised how many people are willing to pitch in!

TIP: Learn to Not Answer the Telephone

Investing in an answering machine or voice mail will also prove to be a boon. Although many people run to answer the phone each time it rings, the lupus patient must carefully apportion his or her energies. You needn't be awakened from a nap, or coaxed into a long conversation before you've had your morning medication. Explain your situation to your loved ones, then turn the ringer off on your phone during those times when you need your rest.

If you work at home, rearrange your workspace so that it doesn't take over the whole house. That way, when you need to rest, you can leave the work in its own place and use your other living areas. Also, arrange your work schedule around lupus as much as possible, so that you can get the full benefit of your rest periods.

Do something nice for your home—and yourself—each week. Perhaps some fresh flowers, a new picture, a new houseplant. Look upon your house or apartment as your home, where you derive the most rest, comfort, and peace. And encourage your family and friends to do the same. You need not hide away from the world—just bring the world, in manageable doses, home to you.

Organization

Simplifying your home life will reduce the stress that you feel, especially when you are in a flare. Streamline your home so that there is less clutter and you know where things are. Keep clear, clean files of your medical records, finances, and other papers, and know where to find them at a moment's notice. Also, keep an updated list of contact telephone numbers handy (taped under the telephone, perhaps, or on a bulletin board beside it). Remember, the less time you spend trying to locate a number or a paper, the more time you will have to move on with your life.

Rearrange Your Home to Make It Lupus-friendly

One of the frequent complaints of lupus patients is pain: pain in the joints, especially the hips, knees, and hands. Sometimes the pain is so severe that walking is impossible and picking up something as simple as a glass is a chore.

As you go about your day, observe where you experience the most pain in relation to the rooms in your apartment or house. Ask yourself questions as you do so, and jot down the answers in your lupus notebook. Take your home room by room; these questions (and some answers) will get you started:

The Kitchen

"I love to cook," says Ann. "But when I was first diagnosed, my hands were so swollen and painful that I couldn't lift pots and pans, let alone plates filled with food. Bending and lifting were hard, too. Finally I rearranged my cupboards to make it easier to reach things and found cookware that weighed a lot less. It's easier to cook, now. I like being able to do something that I enjoy!"

Here are some questions to keep in mind when evaluating your kitchen:

- Have you arranged your kitchen so that you don't have to stoop to reach often-used utensils or cookware? Keeping the lightest items at the higher levels will help reduce strain on your back, neck, and hands. Also, you might want to consider installing racks with hooks set at a comfortable level for often-used pots and pans.
- Do you spare sore hands and wrists by eliminating the need to pick up heavy cookware or utensils? Reducing the number of plates, pots, and pans that you nestle one on top of the other will also help alleviate some of the strain of lifting.

- Are your dishes light enough so that you can lift and carry them easily, even if they are filled with food? Stoneware dishes can be extremely heavy for the lupus patient, especially when filled with food. Likewise, some high-grade pots and pans can be extremely heavy and dangerous to lift, especially if they are hot from the stove or oven. You might have to donate your present cookware to charity (or give it to a relative or friend) and purchase lighter, more manageable items, such as Corelle dishes, which are lightweight and made of hard-to-break glass. Another option is plastic dishware, some of which is very attractive, affordable, and lightweight.

- Are your cooking utensils of the right shape and size so that they make preparing food, opening jars, and storing items easy for you, even on your most flared days? Several manufacturers have developed larger-handled, easy to manipulate cooking utensils. One of these is OXO. Within their Good Grips line, there are vegetable peelers, ladles, jar openers, pepper mills, scissors, even a broom, and all have rubberized, comfort-sensitive grips. These (or other brands with similar design) take stress off of your hand and wrist joints. Good Grips are available at many housewares and hardware stores.

- Do you have heavy cooking mitts nearby to handle hot pots and pans straight from the oven or stove? For many reasons, the lupus patient must be extra careful to avoid cuts, scrapes, and burns. Although you may not be able to avoid them completely, having the proper protective gear in the kitchen is essential. Inspect it frequently and replace it when it shows signs of wear.

- Is there a first-aid kit close to your cooking area, as well as a fire extinguisher? All well-equipped kitchens should have these anyway. But for the lupus patient, they are especially important. Also, be sure you have been trained in the proper way to use a fire extinguisher, and that it is light enough for you to handle.

- If you are sensitive to the cold, are your refrigerator and freezer arranged in such a way so that you don't have to spend much time in front of an open door, exposing your hands and face to the cold? Placing often-used items toward the front and lesser-used items in the rear of the freezer compartment or refrigerator will help take the chill out of finding what you need.

- Do you have gloves to wear when doing dishes? If you have hand problems, slippery dishes can be even more elusive. Sturdy, rubberized cleaning gloves will help you handle them—and save on replacement costs!
- If you keep your medication in the kitchen, do you store it away from sources of light and heat? The kitchen is a popular place to keep medications because so much of it needs to be taken with food. However, most medication is sensitive to extremes in temperature and exposure to light.
- Are you prepared if a sudden bout of the flu or other flare-induced symptoms strike? Keeping comfort foods such as ginger ale, crackers, and canned soup may come in handy in these situations. Be sure to observe the "use by" and "sell by" dates on packages.

TIP: Grocery Shopping If You Take Prednisone

A lupus patient on prednisone for a short period of time must plan ahead so that grocery shopping is done when one's mind is not under the sugar-craving effects of prednisone. This will keep the pantry bare of sugary and starchy products. If you are on prednisone long-term, be sure to grocery shop after you have eaten a meal, instead of when you are hungry.

The Bedroom

"One of my symptoms is extreme fatigue," says Sylvia. "I have to take a nap every day, or I feel miserable. But at first, my bedroom was a mess. There was clutter everywhere, the television was usually on. I'd even do work in bed! Once I took charge of my 'resting space,' I was able to relax and get the most out of my naps. Good sleep makes a huge difference!"

When evaluating your bedroom, ask yourself these questions:

➤*Do you feel comfortable in your bedroom? If you suffer from lupus fatigue, you will spend a great deal of time in your bedroom, resting and sleeping. Make sure that it is a restful* place, with surroundings that are conducive to sleep and re-cuperation. You might find that a television set is more stress-ful than helpful. Or you might find that falling asleep to the sound of music is therapeutic. Adjust the humidity and the temperature so that you are comfortable. Don't be afraid to make your bedroom your sanctuary! In fact, make it just the kind of place you want to go to when fatigue strikes.

➤If you awaken in the middle of the night with vertigo, is your medication close at hand? Do you have a glass of water, a telephone, and your doctor's telephone number nearby, too? Lupus is unpredictable. You may go to bed feeling fine, yet wake up in the morning unable to move—not an ideal situ-ation in which to go looking for your medication, water, and telephone. Keep these within reach, in case you need them.

➤Do you have esophageal reflux (a medical condition where you sometimes regurgitate gastric contents into your esoph-agus), and does it become particularly active at night? Try placing four- to six-inch bricks or blocks of wood under the head of your bed to elevate it. This may assist gravity in doing its part against the effects of esophageal reflux. (Sleeping with more pillows does not have the same effect, however, and may actually cause more abdominal distress.)

The Bathroom

Here are some things to keep in mind when evaluating your bathroom:

➤Do you keep medications in the bathroom? Because bath-rooms can become hot and steamy, keeping most medica-tions in them is not a good idea. You do not want to run the risk of a loss in drug potency. Move your meds to the kitchen or bedroom instead.

➤Is your bathtub slip-proof? Now is the time to make sure that you have the proper bath mats and handholds so that you minimize your risk of falling in the shower or bath. If you should slip and hurt yourself, have a plan for a way to get help. For example, make sure that there is a telephone near the bathroom (but don't take it into the tub!), as well as the telephone numbers of 911 and your physicians (on speed dial, if your telephone has that capability). Also, keep your Medic Alert bracelet or necklace close at hand.

Other Rooms

Now that you have taken a look at the three most used rooms in your house or apartment, do the same kind of assessment of the other rooms.

> ➤*Are they arranged in a lupus-friendly way? That is, do they provide an easy-to-negotiate traffic pattern? Are the items in them easy to lift, move, and use?*
> ➤*Is there a telephone nearby so that you can call for help if necessary?*
> ➤*Is the lighting in your house or apartment lupus-safe? That is, do you have window coverings that will protect you from the sun's rays if you are photosensitive? Heavy curtains or blinds will do, and you might need to draw them only at the most sun-filled part of the day. Having the coverage is key.*

Helpful Services for the Home

Cleaning services, meal-delivery businesses, even "supermarkets on wheels" can make home life easier for the lupus patient. Ask if they will give discounts for the disabled, or pool your shopping lists with two or three friends and divide the single delivery charge among you to save even more.

Other businesses make house calls, too. For example, many computer companies have in-home maintenance agreements. Not having to lug your computer to a store can save you a lot of time and pain, so you should seriously consider such a maintenance agreement.

Dog walkers can tend to your pooch when you aren't feeling up to it, and a gardener can do the bulk of your outdoor work, thus saving you exposure to the sun while maintaining the beauty of your garden. When it comes time to paint the house or do significant remodeling, enlist the services of professional painters and handy people. To locate these or other in-house helpers, ask your neighbors and friends for referrals, or contact your local chamber of commerce, church, or other civic organization.

Unusual Helpers: Pets as Domestic Aides

For those lupus patients who are severely mobility impaired, or who have serious hearing loss or other handicaps, one possible helpmate is a dog. Beyond their sight-assistance capabilities, many dogs are now trained to open doors, pick up telephones, alert their humans when there is someone at the door—even warn them when there is a fire or other problem at home and call 911! Such skills, in addition to their companionship, make these dogs invaluable additions to many households.

Some of these dogs are purebreds, but others come from the local animal shelters. There are agencies and organizations that train dogs for specific duties, and they will also train the dogs' owners to make sure they are handling their canine companions properly. If you feel you could benefit from such assistance, speak with your doctor or a veterinarian and contact your local animal shelter. Some other organizations that may help, too, are listed in the back of this book.

If You Have to Move

Moving can be one of the most traumatic activities you can ever engage in, but sometimes it is necessary due to job relocation, the need to be closer to family members, or even medical necessity, such as need for a climate change. As difficult as it is, however, moving need not be completely painful. Here are some suggestions for making your move a little easier:

When you find out that you have to move, sit down with those involved (your spouse, children, other family, friends) and map out a time line for all the things that need to be done. Ask your spouse or friends to help you take on some of the tasks ahead, and if your children are old enough, give them some things to do, too. At regular intervals, hold family meetings to talk about the progress of plans. Use these times to discuss personal concerns, too, and the positive aspects of embarking on a new adventure.

Moving companies can be helpful, too, particularly if you are relocating a large household a great distance. Tell your mover about your constraints, and work with the staff to take some of the burden off of your shoulders.

Adapting to the Demands of Medication and Discomfort

Living with lupus involves planning ahead and staying organized so that you have enough energy to lead a productive life. Conserve energy by avoiding walking or climbing a lot of stairs as you go about your daily tasks. Activities that require more endurance or more cognitive abilities should be done at a time of day when these capabilities are at their best.

Muscle weakness and weight gain may occur as a consequence of the disease or as side effects of medication. Training with ankle and arm weights or an exercise video can help offset these handicaps and also help to get around prohibitions against being outside in the sun or in bad weather. Hot baths, paraffin baths, and light massages are good nonmedicinal ways of treating pain in the joints and muscles. One can prevent excessive strain on one's muscles and joints by using a cart to carry an otherwise heavy handbag or groceries.

Regular sleep is important for proper secretion and rhythm of many important hormones and nerve-messenger substances. It is important to wind down in the evening so that one's mind is conducive to falling asleep. The sleep environment must be quiet, dark, and at a comfortable temperature. If a spouse snores at night, it may be important to discuss this with his or her doctor and obtain help for this problem.

If you have esophageal reflux, avoid eating chocolate and drinking alcohol and caffeinated beverages, as these can worsen reflux. Lying down or sleeping within two hours of eating can also increase the chances of acid secretions flowing backward into your esophagus and throat. Reflux of acid may be an important cause of a dry cough, wheezing, recurrent sinus congestion, and throat and ear pain.

Check into the particulars of your health plan and try to line up a primary-care physician before you move. You might even call that doctor and introduce yourself before your first official appointment.

If you have more latitude in choosing your own physician, ask your doctor for referrals in your new area. Call those referrals and, if possible, visit with those doctors before moving. Knowing you have set up your medical team, at least partially, will give you tremendous peace of mind as you tend to other aspects of your relocation. And be sure to keep a copy of all your medical records so that your new physician can be brought up to speed on your lupus history and current treatments and symptoms.

Through all the upheaval of a move, don't ignore the fact that you have lupus! Unfortunately, lupus does not go away simply because we want it to. In fact, it is in just those stressful kinds of situations when lupus can flare. Keep in contact with your doctor, continue to follow his or her instructions, and take extra time to rest. That way, you can be more prepared to enjoy your new living situation when you actually settle in.

13

THE PERSONAL FACTOR:

Having a Life

There is a world outside of lupus. Investigating that world will help you through some of your daily struggles with the disease. Having activities and hobbies that you look forward to and that make you feel excited about life does much to keep the wolf at bay. Although you may find that you are forced to give up some hobbies or other activities that you used to enjoy, your life with lupus can still be a full one. Indeed, investigating this new world will undoubtedly lead to surprising discoveries of people, places, and activities that you might not have found out about if you had not been diagnosed with lupus. And, while it may be a challenge at times to get yourself where you want to go or be, there are resources to assist the lupus patient around the home and ways to deal with circumstances outside the home.

Hobbies and Activities

When you are in the throes of a flare, you might want to take up a new hobby or activity that you can do at home, at your own pace. Perhaps there is something you've always wanted to learn or do. Now is the time to do it. And you might find surprising physical benefits from certain activities.

Alternatives
You might also be able to find enjoyable alternatives related to those you used to enjoy, thus enabling yourself to keep a hand in something you really like to do. Here are some suggestions:

- Instead of swimming outdoors, try aquatic exercise in an indoor pool, which will protect you from the sun's harmful rays.
- If you used to play tennis, try badminton, Ping-Pong, or gentle racquetball to lessen the strain on your joints.
- You may not be able to play golf during the day anymore; however, you can still play night golf, pitch and putt, or virtual golf indoors.
- Crowded public events might be prohibitive if you have a tendency to catch contagious infections. You can adapt to this new restriction by joining a local museum or aquarium and taking advantage of their smaller "for members only" activities.
- Outdoor gardening can be difficult for you during the day, but many lupus patients still maintain their landscape by gardening at night. Still others exercise their green thumbs by tending indoor houseplants.
- If your lupus causes you to stop working, you can find alternative ways to exercise your mind and keep in touch with others. Joining a book club or reading group can help, as can becoming part of a collectors' group.

Hidden Benefits

Some activities might help you cope with specific physical and emotional effects of lupus.

- Joint-friendly movement with music (e.g., ballroom dancing) can keep you limber and help you feel more attractive.
- Needlework, woodworking, or piano playing can help maintain your finger dexterity.
- Chess playing or bridge can help broaden your group of friends while keeping your mind alert.
- A Bible study or other activity with a faith community can help you grow spiritually and make new friends, too.

Dream!

Perhaps there is something you've always wanted to learn or do. Now is the time to figure out how to do it. Having lupus doesn't mean that you have to stop dreaming. With careful consideration, talking with others, and keeping your dream in mind and heart, you can find a way!

Getting around Town

You may not realize it at first, but lupus and its debilitating symptoms enable you to avail yourself of certain special accommodations. When you are out and about, driving, shopping, or enjoying a night on the town, these accommodations can make your life much easier.

Handicap parking placards, for example, relieve you of the need to walk long, painful distances to and from your destination. They also cut down on the amount of time you spend outdoors, going from your car to your destination and back again.

Likewise, handicap access for entrances, rest rooms, and other venues makes it easy for you to arrive at your destination without waiting in lines and aggravating your condition.

If you plan to attend a large function at a public arena or stadium, inquire about handicap seating, which is usually easier to reach and more spacious than some of the more cramped, hard-to-access general seats. Do not plan to pay less for this seating, but do expect to be more comfortable and secure while enjoying the event.

Restaurants and Gatherings

When you make reservations to eat out, request a table indoors, away from bright sunlight, and as far away from smoking as possible. It might surprise you, but some restaurants place their smoking and nonsmoking sections right next to each other, and the smoke can travel to your area quite easily. Also, ask the waiter to indicate special requests on your order. If you encounter resistance to any of your requests, explain that you are asking for such accommodation because of a serious medical condition. Sometimes you might want to carry your own salad dressing, other condiments, bottled water, or decaffeinated tea bag, too, so that you can flavorfully and healthfully enjoy your food.

Private gatherings where people are smoking or coughing and sneezing from illness, or that are out-of-doors, are more problematic for the lupus patient. On the one hand, you do not want to alienate yourself from others. You want—and should enjoy—a social life! But on the other hand, you are correct in not exposing yourself to things that can do you harm.

It is important that you do not let down your guard, even for just one time. All it takes is one sunburn, one exposure to something that's going around, one night spent breathing in smoke, to throw your health off balance or even do you serious harm. You are better off excusing yourself politely, and explaining that you would love to spend time with your friends, but that you cannot risk illness or other damage to your health. A good friend will understand and support you in your desire to maintain your health.

Weddings and Other Rites of Passage

While some plans can be canceled or put off, many human "rites of passage" cannot. You cannot, for example, stop someone from turning a year older. You cannot, in most instances, postpone or cancel a wedding because you suddenly go into a flare (unless you are the bride or groom). And you certainly have no control over when an emergency happens to someone you love, or when someone dies.

In these cases, you should try to do as much as you can to be involved in your loved ones' events, while still taking all the precautions you need to for your health. You can also prepare in advance for some things and thus be ready when events occur. One lupus patient, for example, on shopping trips when she is feeling well, purchases things she sees that would make good gifts throughout the year. This is especially useful when she is in a flare and does not have the energy to go out and buy a gift.

Buying greeting cards in advance is another way to prepare for events, as is keeping a current list of florists, candy stores, and gift services that will allow you to order items over the telephone or Internet in case you cannot get out to purchase them. Keeping some wrapping paper, tape, and ribbon on hand is helpful, too, as is starting Christmas, Hanukkah, and other holiday shopping early so that you're not running around at the last minute.

If you are included in the wedding party, or are asked to participate in other ceremonies or events, explain that a flare might prevent you from being there, and help the person who asks you to participate to come up with a contingency plan. You will feel much better if you cannot go through with what you are asked to do, and your friend or relative will feel better, too.

Travel

Troy has been to Australia, Europe, and many places in the United States. He also suffers from severe, organ-involving lupus. On a trip to Hong Kong, his lupus flared, and he ended up in the hospital. But this hasn't stopped him from further world exploration.

"There isn't anywhere I won't think of going," says Troy, who has had lupus since he was a teenager. "Sometimes I just take extra precautions. For instance, I know I have problems at high altitudes. If I'm going skiing, I'll just leave a day early and get acclimated before I go out on the slopes."

Once you are diagnosed with lupus, your whole perception of leaving home to take a trip changes. Suddenly you worry about whether you'll go into a flare while you are away from your immediate support system or, worse, that you will develop new or unusual symptoms or suffer an accident away from your regular medical team. You find the extra load you must carry (medications, lupus-friendly clothing and accessories, hot pads, etc.) too heavy to seem feasible. And you wonder, with all the extra baggage you must take, if you will indeed enjoy your trip or if it will merely be more of a stressful headache.

Provided your health is stable, you can still plan to travel, within certain parameters. When you make your travel arrangements, do everything you can to accommodate your medical condition, and take the extra precaution of purchasing emergency travel insurance, if you feel the need. If you have to cancel your plans, do so with grace, accepting that sometimes lupus intervenes, and knowing that there will be a time when it will not, and your plans can proceed uninterrupted.

Before You Go

In the early stages of planning a trip:

> *Talk with your doctor about where you want to go and how you will get there and back. He or she might suggest alternative destinations or methods of travel. For example, your rheumatologist might not think you are up to a twelve-hour car ride, but you could get to the same place by airplane with little or no difficulty.*

➤Investigate the medical facilities and/or health-care system in the place you want to go. A third-world country with questionable hygienic practices or less modern medical facilities is a disaster waiting to happen for a person with a compromised immune system.

➤Decide how you will get there. Do you want to take a tour or be on your own? Do you want to rent a car at your destination, or rely on public transportation or walking? If you opt for a tour, try to select one that does not have you on the go every day, but allows for a few days in one place so that you can get your bearings, sightsee, and still have a chance to tend to your health.

➤What kinds of activities will you want to participate in, and what impact will these have on your need for rest?

➤If you need special accommodations, make sure that you will have no problems with them before you pay your deposit; it is a good idea to get special requests confirmed in writing so there is no confusion down the road.

➤Get a complete checkup before you embark upon your trip.

➤If you need to have your joints injected, do so before your trip.

➤Ask your doctor for a letter outlining your current medical condition, list of medications you are taking, and any special considerations regarding your health, in case you need emergency medical attention.

➤Get at least one referral for a rheumatologist in the area to which you will travel before you go, and utilize it if you encounter problems.

➤Learn some medical words in the language of the place to which you are going so that you can communicate your health symptoms clearly, if need be.

Insurance for Traveling

Research health insurance and travel/trip insurance before you go, and make sure you are covered if you need medical attention abroad. Check with your own medical plan to know exactly what you are covered for in the area you are planning to visit. If you are covered by a health maintenance organization (HMO), also verify that you can receive medical attention if you are elsewhere in the

TIP: Get a Medic Alert Bracelet

Whether you travel around your hometown or abroad, you should wear a medical bracelet or necklace and carry a wallet card indicating your need for immediate medical attention in case of accident. Some services, such as Medic Alert (www.medicalert.com), will provide you with these and a service whereby the person assisting you can call an 800 number and find out who your primary physician is, what your current medications are, and any allergies or unusual conditions you might have. Although you might think you don't need this extra protection, think about what would happen if you are knocked unconscious and cannot answer for yourself. How will the medical response team know what to do for you? And if they guess, what will happen if they guess inappropriately?

United States, and find out exactly what you need to do (precertify care, etc.) prior to receiving such care.

If you feel you need extra coverage, speak with your travel agent or tour operator. Your travel agent, the American Automobile Association, or tour operator can also help you with acquiring international medical insurance. With many policies, there is a clause dealing with preexisting conditions, so make sure you know all the parameters of your chosen plan before you travel.

Travel (or trip) protection insurance will usually reimburse your non-reimbursed travel expenses if an emergency occurs right before or during your trip, causing it to be canceled, interrupted, or delayed. There are a number of circumstances covered by the insurance, and these can vary from policy to policy. Again, be sure you know all that your policy covers before paying the premium.

Because many hospitals and clinics in other countries require you to pay your fees up front, be sure that you have some way of providing a significant payment should the need arise. You might also want to consider purchasing a just-in-case policy with an emergency evacuation service, such as MedJet (www.medjetassistance.com), which will transport you by private jet back to the United States and your home doctor, in case you cannot get appropriate care away from home.

Luggage and Other Equipment

You will need to make sure that your luggage supports you on your trip. It should have easy-grip handles (ones that are cushioned and wide enough to alleviate aggravating your hand discomfort). Also, each piece, from the carry-on to the garment bag, should be on wheels, preferably ones that are partially recessed into the bag itself (wheels that protrude are too prone to getting caught on escalators or breaking off due to baggage handling or usual wear and tear). Although you might have people carting your luggage for you during a good portion of your trip, there will still be times when you will have to move it or lift it, and the easier it is to maneuver, the better.

You should plan to pack as lightly as possible. If you are going to be gone awhile, or need heavier clothing, think about sending a box

TIP: Take All Crucial Items On Board in Carry-on Luggage

Never check medications, wigs, or other lupus-related devices in your luggage. Carry it all onto the plane in your carry-on. If you need two carry-ons, take two carry-ons. And if you encounter trouble with the ground crew or flight attendants who want you to check one bag, explain that the carry-ons contain essential medical equipment for your disability. Such items are almost always exempt from baggage carry-on restrictions. If you are nervous about relying on your own explanation for your load, get your doctor to write a letter explaining your situation.

If you don't want to carry all your medical items in your carry-ons, consider that none of them will be covered or reimbursed by the airline if your luggage is lost. And you will find yourself doing without the very things that make healthy travel possible!

ahead to your destination instead of trying to pack everything into your luggage.

What to Pack

Besides the usual items that you always take with you on the road, there are some specific, lupus-related things that you will need.

You should take all your medicines in their original containers, as well as extras in case you drop a pill or need to increase your dosage while away. Also, you should check with your doctor to see if he or she wants you to take a supply of antibiotics or other medications just in case. Some prescription insurance plans allow you to obtain extra medication beyond your regularly prescribed quantities. This is called a vacation refill, and your pharmacist can help you if you need one.

Pack a small first-aid kit with your carry-on, as well as a packet of moist towelettes, which come in very handy if you cannot get to a rest room to wash your hands. Take a good-sized bottle of water on the plane or train, and make sure you drink from it frequently to keep yourself hydrated.

Take your lupus-friendly clothing, extra sunscreen, and a good pair of sunglasses (or two, if you tend to lose them). Even if it is winter where you are going, the glare of the sun can bring you discomfort. Consider taking anything else that helps sustain your health, but if it is very bulky or unwieldy (for example, a favorite set of pillows), use your creativity to determine whether you can improvise comfortably while on the road.

Assistance along the Way

At airports, train stations, and some bus terminals, porters can ease your luggage woes. Flag one down as soon as you arrive, or call ahead to make arrangements to have someone meet you at the entrance. Airport porters can take your bags to the ticket counter and help you with your carry-ons up to the gate. At the train station, they can go all the way onto the train and put your bags into the storage area. Tip these helpful people and be very pleasant—they can make your trip flow much, much easier. Ask, too, if you can have assistance in putting your carry-ons into the overhead compartments. Sometimes cabin attendants are hesitant to do this, but if you have requested such a service in advance, the airline might find someone else to help you instead.

In airports, many airlines have a separate handicap lounge,

staffed with customer service agents and equipped with a rest room, flight monitors, and comfortable seating. If your flight is delayed or canceled, you can seek assistance at the handicap lounge, rather than wait in long lines at ticket counters or gates. Usually the handicap lounge is not advertised, so be sure to ask an airline employee where it is when you arrive at the airport.

Because many lupus patients do not manifest their disease externally, it is sometimes helpful to carry a cane with you if you will be traveling long distances, especially at peak travel times. Or, if you have severe hand involvement, wear a brace on one or both arms. Such a visible sign of physical problems can make it easier for other people to understand and comply with your request for accommodation or help.

When You Arrive

The saying, "When you go on vacation, lupus takes a vacation" is simply not true. Lupus is with you all day, every day, and you will have to take precautions while you travel, just as you would at home. You need to make time for rest and stretches or other exercise, and you need to maintain as healthy a diet as possible. You should take your medication on schedule and keep a faithful symptom log on the road, too.

Besides the "normal" things you must do, traveling can pose other challenges that will need your attention. These include changes in time zones and/or climate, to which your body must acclimate, the stress of being in a strange place and not having your support system readily available, perhaps even the sensation of being totally lost because of language, cultural, or other barriers. Be aware of these challenges and gauge how you will react to them. Be patient with yourself and the world around you. This will help you cope with the frustrations of traveling and help you see the wonders of a new place with fresh, excited eyes.

How to Choose the Right Time and the Right Way to Travel If You Have Lupus

Lupus patients with arthritis and severe autonomic symptoms such as Raynaud's phenomenon, dry eyes and dry mouth, irritable bowel syndrome, and migraine headache often do not feel well with sudden changes in temperature and barometric pressure. Hence it is best to travel to a place where the weather is relatively stable and is not subject to sudden changes.

If a patient has organ involvement, such as impaired gas exchange due to lung disease, special precautions must be taken with an oxygen prescription test prior to flying in an airplane that is pressurized with a lower oxygen tension than room air. A dialysis center must be located prior to traveling to the new location if a patient has kidney failure.

Infections can flare up because of lupus; hence, precautions to avoid food- and water-borne illnesses must be taken. It is preferable to have only bottled drinks and food that is served hot if the patient is not certain about the potability of the tap water used to wash vegetables or fruit. Fruit that may be peeled is generally safe to eat, although lupus patients with irritable bowel syndrome are often very sensitive to unexpected food items, and hence it is preferable to stay with food that the person knows will agree with him or her.

Vaccinations against hepatitis A and B, typhoid, cholera, and pneumonia should be undertaken when appropriate. Hydroxychloroquine often suffices for malaria prophylaxis except in areas endemic for resistant Falciparum malaria, in which case other agents such as mefloquine or proguanil should be used. Live vaccinations for yellow fever, dengue, chicken pox, rabies, measles, mumps, rubella or polio are relatively contraindicated in lupus patients, especially if they are on immunosuppressive agents, and travel to endemic areas should be avoided.

14

THE PERSONAL FACTOR:

Looking Great Even When You Feel Awful

You will fight lupus only as effectively as you take care of yourself. And you will take care of yourself the best when you feel good about yourself. So you must pay close attention to all areas of your personal life—exercise, appearance, and grooming—to make sure that you take care of them well.

Exercise

Find and maintain a comfortable and regular level of exercise. Although certain joint involvement and other symptoms might restrict the types of exercise lupus patients can engage in, most lupus patients can and should exercise. This will ensure sustained muscle tone, heart strength, and better lung function, and bring you a sense of accomplishment.

Pam Leitner, a physical therapist, says, "You need to find someone who understands autoimmune disease. The Arthritis Foundation has some fabulous programs, and some hospitals have recreation programs."

When you find a qualified professional to help you tailor an exercise program, Leitner suggests you keep these things in mind:

• Set personal, reachable goals in small-step increments
• Exercise with a buddy if you don't like to do it alone

- Give yourself some leeway; don't try to be perfect
- Establish activities that you can do even on the days when you do not feel like exercising fully—some exercises can be effective even when done sitting in a chair

"With exercise, you have to be self-motivated," says Leitner. "But you don't have to think you have to sweat and get your heart rate up all the time. Work around the house or around the yard. Find movement opportunities. Listen to your body and start slowly. And don't be a weekend warrior! Try to do only half of what you think you can do and be sure to stop before you get any pain."

Because each lupus patient is different, each patient should consult his or her doctor to find out what constitutes prudent exercise in his or her case. A referral to a physical therapist can also assist you in finding a level of exercise that is appropriate and effective.

Diet

There is no "lupus diet" designed to cure or curtail the disease. However, there are guidelines for eating that can alleviate some of the complications from lupus and the medications used to treat it.

One of the most serious problems lupus patients face is the tendency toward heart disease and heart attacks. Much of this is due to the prednisone that many patients must take. But much is also due to a poor diet and to untreated chronic inflammation in the blood.

You can reduce your chances of developing heart problems by decreasing your fat and sodium intake and increasing the amount of fresh fruits and vegetables that you consume. If you have kidney disease, it is especially important that you reduce your salt intake, as well as protein (0.6 to 0.8 gram per kilo of your body weight is the guideline for daily protein consumption).

Weight

If you eat nutritionally and exercise, you should be able to maintain a healthy weight. However, certain factors can influence you to overeat, become listless, or consume foods that are laden with fat, sugar, and salt.

• Prednisone

One of the myths of prednisone is that you will always gain weight when you take it. Although it is true that your appetite and craving for carbohydrates can increase, especially if you take high doses of it, prednisone need not make you gain weight if you carefully watch your intake of sugar, salt, fat, and carbohydrates *and* stay active while on it.

• Depression

Emotions play a key role in being able to cope with lupus. If you become depressed, you might turn to bingeing on non-nutritional foods, and you might become inactive. Discuss your emotional response to lupus with your doctor and your support group and your lupus buddy. A referral to a therapist can help you sort through your feelings and put them into perspective. Sometimes medication can be beneficial in helping you battle depression.

• Joint Pain

If you suffer from joint pain, you might be inclined to stop moving. This, in turn, could cause you to gain weight and lose muscle tone and stamina. Although lupus patients with joint involvement should avoid many forms of weight-bearing exercise, there are programs designed for people with certain limitations. The Arthritis Foundation has one such program called PACE (People with Arthritis Can Exercise.) Local chapters of the Arthritis Foundation often offer several PACE classes, as do some YMCAs, community centers, and exercise and dance studios. Some forms of yoga can be helpful to maintaining flexibility. Good old-fashioned walking is another easy and pleasant way to go! The important thing about all these activities is to keep yourself moving. Do what you can when you are in a flare and work to gain more strength when you feel better. Your body will be stronger for it!

• Fatigue

Sometimes when you are tired, the last thing you want to do is cook a nutritious meal. The temptation to stop at a local fast-food restaurant can be overwhelming. Plan ahead, however, and prepare food in advance and freeze it so you won't have to cook when you are greatly fatigued and in pain. Purchase ready-chopped packages of vegetables and salads so that you can save your sore hands the work of preparing them yourself.

Appearance

Lupus can affect your personal appearance by bringing on rashes and hair loss, not to mention a "blah" feeling. You can combat the sense that you are doing poorly (which can weigh you down significantly) by taking special care with your appearance, trying new clothing styles, and adding fashion accents to your wardrobe that will brighten your mood and detract from your ill health. Even on a tight budget, it is possible to add one splash of color, one new item of clothing, and rejuvenate your tired spirits.

"You're sick? I don't believe it. You look so good!"

Each person with lupus will hear these words, probably more than once, and feel a twisting, uncomfortable twinge in the pit of his or her stomach. The urge to snap back will be strong. The need to set the person straight will be overwhelming.

In a way, not looking as bad as you feel is not such a terrible thing. In fact, it is probably *better* that your face doesn't reflect what's happening inside your body! And if you do have physical manifestations of lupus, there are things you can do to lessen their visibility and bring back some of the self-esteem that you might lose as a result of them.

Hair Loss

Hair loss (alopecia) due to lupus can happen strand by strand or clump by clump. You might notice evidence of it in your shower drain or hairbrush, or fistfuls of hair might pull completely out of your scalp. Many women (and men) put great emphasis on their hair care, using expensive hair-care products, beauty salon treatments, and adornments. When hair falls out, a woman can feel severely traumatized that part of her identity is being lost. A man might fear he is losing his attractiveness and, possibly, his virility.

Once you have lost enough hair for it to be noticeable, you might explore several options to mitigate the loss and regain some of your lost self-esteem.

Medical Treatments

Your rheumatologist or dermatologist can suggest several medical treatments that might or might not work to regenerate hair growth, depending on the cause of your hair loss. These include cortisone

Causes for Hair Loss in SLE

About 50 percent of women with lupus experience severe hair loss that is sometimes not reversible. This has significant effects on the person's self-esteem and her ability to cope with other life-threatening aspects of her illness. The causes for hair loss in lupus are protean and range from disease-specific to medication-induced.

The disease itself may cause hair loss in multiple ways. Immune activity may destroy the hair follicles, arrest growth of the hair, and result in regional loss of hair called alopecia areata in a small part of the scalp, or may cause more extensive hair loss in a larger part of the scalp. These hair follicles may be salvaged and allowed to grow with local injections of steroids. A more serious and permanent scarring rash, called a discoid rash, may result in permanent hair loss in the affected area, and needs to be treated urgently with antimalarial drugs to prevent its progression.

Other autoimmune illnesses, such as decreased thyroid hormone production, can also result in hair loss. Severe anemia, which is a decrease in the number of oxygen-carrying cells in the blood, may also cause hair loss. In fact, any serious organ-threatening illness due to lupus or infections can cause a reversible shedding of the hair called telogen effluvium. The hair goes through its normal rest cycle of three to six months all at once and then grows up. Hair follicle roots can be seen clearly in this condition, indicating that the hair will return.

Medications used to treat lupus, such as methotrexate and cyclophosphamide, which are chemotherapy medicines, will cause hair loss. Other medications, such as hydroxychloroquine (an antimalarial) and steriods, cause hair loss less often. It is often difficult to understand whether the hair loss after a severe disease flare is due to the illness causing telogen effluvium, which is reversible, or is the result of a new medication that is started to treat the disease flare. In general, examining for the presence of hair roots in the balding area and being patient for three to six months to see if the hair will come back can help differentiate between the two possible causes.

injections, creams and gels, and other medications. Sometimes, however, hair loss is a direct result of the autoimmune process and cannot be curtailed except through treatment for the lupus, which could take a great deal of time. In this case, you will need to find other, more cosmetic ways of "covering up" for the loss.

Wigs, Falls, and Extensions

Exploring these options need not be as traumatic as you might think. For one thing, you could change your whole look with the simple addition of a wig that is a different color, length, or style from your real hair. You could also purchase more than one wig to give yourself options, depending on your mood or the clothes you plan to wear on any given day.

Wig wearing can relieve you of the stress of styling your own hair each day—with so many of the new and improved styles that are wash and wear, there will be no more bad-hair days! And caring for wigs is so easy that you will spend much less time fussing over expensive shampoos, mousses, and conditioners.

Choosing the right wig is, of course, important. You will find them available through mail-order companies and in costume shops or stores exclusively devoted to wigs and other hairpieces. Here are some tips for choosing a wig:

- Shop for a wig with a friend to get a trusted second opinion. Also bring a hat, because some wigs are so thick that they can't be comfortably worn with hats.
- Try on several styles, checking for ease of flow, naturalness, and the flatter factor (how well the wig flatters you).
- Pay close attention to comfort of fit; you will be wearing your wig throughout the day, and want it to sit securely but comfortably on your head.
- Comparison shop to find the right price for the wig you want—natural-hair wigs are more expensive than synthetic, and not necessarily better.
- Select a wig that you can wash at home and that will retain its style through repeated washings.
- Understand the warranty and return policies for whatever wig you purchase.
- A fall is a hairpiece that attaches to a scarf or other item and drapes down from it. Extensions are woven directly onto your existing hair. While both can look very natural and stylish, keep in mind that weaving extensions onto already

fragile hair could be disastrous. More of your hair could fall out before the autoimmune process is under control. A wig is the best course of action for you, unless you are sure that your existing hair can support other alternatives.

When you first wear your wig, friends will notice that you are wearing it. But when it comes to strangers noticing how great your hair looks, you do not need to explain. Simply smile and say "Thank you"—and mean it!

Further Support

Talking with other lupus patients who are coping with hair loss can ease your fears and give you more creative suggestions about how to deal with it. Also, the National Alopecia Foundation (www.naaf.org) is an excellent source of information on the latest in hair-loss treatments, research, and support.

Rashes and Makeup

Lupus rashes can be aggravating, unsightly, and very shocking to you and other people. Your doctor can help you find a medical course of action to treat them, but you might also want to explore cosmetic ways of concealing them when they flare. This can actually be a fun thing to do (remember playing dress-up as a child?), and helps boost your self-esteem at a time when it could be seriously damaged.

Skin Products

Before you try any creams or oils on your face or body, take the list of ingredients to your doctor to verify that you can use the product safely. Some additives, such as tea tree oil, can be irritating to the lupus patient. Others, especially those containing alpha hydroxy-butyric acid, might cause secondary rashes or allergic reactions that might then require additional medical treatment.

Makeup

For the lupus patient with facial rashes, less makeup is probably better than more. Select a shade of base that will tone down the redness of your skin without looking like a caked mask. Try to find a product that contains sunblock as well, or that is light enough so that you can comfortably apply a sunblock over it.

Spread the base evenly, remembering to blend it up to your hairline and down your neck. If you have a malar (butterfly) rash or other redness on the cheeks, you might not need blush. If you use rouge or other coloration, be sure to do so subtly.

Eye makeup can be irritating, especially if you have Sjögren's syndrome, which can dry out your eyes and affect your eyelids. If you choose to use eye makeup anyway, select hypoallergenic products that are light and moist.

Medications and Sjögren's can cause dryness in and around the mouth. Keep a tube of lip balm handy and use it liberally throughout the day and before bed. Moist lipsticks are preferred over dry pencils.

Sun Sensitivity

Many lupus patients already know they are sensitive to the sun. Others don't know it yet, but might develop such sensitivity over time. It is a good idea to err on the side of being cautious, particularly because the sun can exacerbate lupus symptoms and bring on flares without much warning.

TIP: Take Vitamin D

One of the adverse effects of avoiding sunlight is that vitamin D synthesis in the skin is inhibited, since this is dependent on sunlight exposure. At least 400 IU of vitamin D, which is the average daily requirement, must be supplemented in the diet.

A Sun-sensitive Awareness

You might not think that you expose yourself to the sun all that much. Perhaps you go only from the house to the car to the office and back home again. But if you really thought about it, you would realize that the sun (and the rays that penetrate the clouds on an overcast day) still reaches your exposed skin. It comes in through the windows of your car; it lights your way from the car to the office. If you take a walk at lunchtime, you expose yourself to sun then. And your trip home is affected in the same way as your trip to work.

As you go about your daily activities, gauge the times when you are outside, even in your car. You will be surprised at how much you come into contact with the sun's rays—and how much you need to be conscientious about applying sunscreen and using other precautions to avoid exposure.

Essentials

To protect yourself from the sun, you will need several things:

• Hats

Select hats with at least a three-and-a-half- to four-inch brim all the way around the crown of the hat. Make sure they are made from dense material (avoid the thinner straw variety that allow the sun to enter through).

• Sun-protective Clothing

There are several companies today that manufacture UV-protective clothing of various styles, colors, and prices. A list of some of those companies is included at the back of this book. You need not change your whole wardrobe, however. Some of the best sun protection is probably already in your closet! When you are out in the sun, wear long-sleeved, dense shirts, or combine tank tops with a pull-on long-sleeved shirt or jacket. Make sure that your neck is protected, too—either select clothing with a high neckline, or wrap a scarf around the area that is exposed. Wear pants or skirts that cover your legs thoroughly, and don't forget stockings or socks to cover your ankles, too. Gloves can also be useful, particularly if you will be driving (think of the sun streaming through the windshield and hitting your sensitive hands). As with your selection of hats, pick out clothing that expresses who you are; don't feel as though you have to be mummified in camouflage. Use this new clothing opportunity as a chance to really express yourself, your sense of humor, and your innate attractiveness.

• Sunscreen

There are many products on the market that profess to provide adequate protection against the UV-A and UV-B rays of the sun. However, not all of these products will work for you.

Finding the right sunscreen might take some trial and error. Here are some tips:

* Know your skin type and predisposition to tanning and burning before you purchase a sunscreen.
* A higher SPF is not necessarily better. An "SPF" (Sun Protection Factor) of 15 is generally high enough to protect most people.
* Scents and fancy colors are not important. You will need to wear sunscreen *every* time you go out. This means that you will wear it to the market, to work, to school, even to the doctor's office.
* Avoid sunscreens that carry a potent smell or that have odd tints that can make your face appear more like a Halloween mask than the real you.
* A waterproof sunscreen is important, but not essential. If you live in a very hot and humid climate during the summer, you might find it easier to keep sunscreen on if it is waterproof.
* Apply sunscreen approximately two hours before going out, and put it on over your makeup, even if it is a cloudy day (harmful rays can penetrate the clouds, even through the rain). Reapply it every six hours, or more frequently if necessary.
* Keep a bottle in the car and one in your purse, as well as one at home. That way you'll have it handy when you need it.

Well-meaning, but Aggravating

When you feel rotten, but look well, how can you respond to others' comments about your great appearance with grace instead of grit?

Never feel as though you need to apologize or offer any excuses for your disease. When someone compliments your appearance, say, "Thank you." When someone remarks on your lovely new hairstyle, and you know you are really wearing a wig, say, "Thank you." When someone oohs and ahhs and asks you where you got that wonderful hat, tell them. And say, "Thank you."

Looking great is really a blessing, and something to be thankful for—with a smile!

How Much Sun Exposure Is OK and What Can Be Done to Avoid Flares Due to Sunlight?

Experiments done with controlled exposure to ultraviolet have shown that both the UV-A and UV-B components of sunlight are capable of causing a flare-up of lupus. Sunlight appears to damage DNA within the skin cells, exposing concealed proteins from within the nucleus of cells to an immune system that is overactive due to lupus. Such experiments have shown that sunlight may cause both skin and internal organ flares in lupus patients.

Sunrises and sunsets appear beautiful and rosy red because only the red component of light, which has the longest wavelength, is not bent away from the earth due to refraction during the early morning and late evening. Harmful ultraviolet light with the shortest wavelength is lost from sunlight due to the longer distances it has to travel in the earth's atmosphere. If they must do so out-of-doors, lupus patients should exercise or swim during the early-morning and early evening hours between six A.M. and eight A.M. and six P.M. and eight P.M., approximately. This is because the most harmful ultraviolet light is at its weakest at those times.

Patients with lupus differ in their sensitivities to sunlight and must take appropriate precautions. Some people may be able to get by with skin creams with an SPF of 15. Other patients require hats, clothing that covers them entirely, or special clothing that reflects sunlight away from them.

15

The Relationship Factor

There are few things more important to the lupus patient than the relationships he or she nurtures. Having close friends upon whom you can rely, and being a friend in return, is the greatest gift of life, exceeding all store-bought possessions. So, too, is having a family, immediate and/or extended, that is supportive, uplifting, and strong.

The quality of your relationships will determine the quality of your life in so many ways. Good friends share the good times and extend helping hands when you need them; a good marriage can provide a haven from pain and suffering and contribute to your sense of belonging in the world; and children can be a blessing to you in youth, as well as in old age. New acquaintances and friendships, relationships that are forged out of your life with lupus, will also be good medicine if approached and nurtured well.

Relationships and Lupus

Any illness can be a lonely experience. But a chronic illness can be particularly isolating. When you are not feeling well, you will have to rest, possibly skipping events that would put you in contact with people you love. Also, there is the need to avoid infection; at certain times of the year (particularly during flu season), you need to take extra precautions to avoid crowds, where you might be exposed to potent germs that could wreak havoc with your immune system.

Having lupus also makes you different from many other people. Misunderstandings or lack of information might prompt others to avoid you out of unfounded fears of contagion.

Paula says, "I remember one time very clearly. I was introduced to someone and sat beside her. During the course of the conversation, I told her I have lupus. She got this horrified look on her face and actually moved her chair so that she was no longer sitting next to me."

Of course, you know that lupus is not contagious. But it will take much more work to turn public awareness around so that everyone else knows the same thing.

Depression can also cause you to isolate yourself from people. The profound sense of loss and sorrow can weigh so heavily upon you that you do not feel like going out or socializing. But it is precisely at these times that contact with others, especially supportive friends and family, is most important.

Reaching Out

Why is it important to maintain relationships with people?

Human beings are social creatures. We live in communities, and work and play with others. Even if we are driving by ourselves on a highway, we are in the company of others who are also driving. People are all around us. Relationships are as natural as breathing.

When you have lupus, however, you need to work harder at developing and maintaining relationships. The illness that can isolate you also makes it difficult for you to be consistent in your social commitments, limits the kinds of activities in which you can participate, and sometimes makes you moody because of the illness or the medication you take to combat it.

To successfully build and maintain relationships, you will need to view them with a different set of "glasses"—ones that allow for the limitations and changes that your lupus brings. And you have to be prepared for rejection and for old friends and even loved ones being unable to cope with your disease.

You have to be prepared to embrace, but you also have to be prepared to let go.

The Perfect Relationship . . .

. . . does not exist!

Still, many relationships can be mutually uplifting, supportive, and joy-inspiring. And relationships where one or both people have lupus are no exceptions.

Here are some characteristics of a positive, healthy relationship:

- The relationship is in balance, with both parties feeling mutual support, affirmation, and trust. Sometimes in a less-than-ideal relationship, one person drains the other of energy and emotional strength. A lupus patient needs to be aware that he or she can ill afford this type of interaction.
- Communication is open and flows consistently from one person to the other. You should feel comfortable talking about your feelings of pain and fear, as well as listening to those of your friend or family member. You must be able to trust that the other person will not put you down because of perceived weaknesses, but will lend a sympathetic ear—and you should do the same. There should always be honesty between you.
- Respect for each other's time and the need to set boundaries is observed by both parties. A true friend will not insist that you do anything that might jeopardize your health or safety.
- Rivalry is at a minimum, with each party respecting the other's talents and accomplishments without being deprecating or jealous. Because of lupus, you might have to pare back your hours at work, or take a position with fewer responsibilities. You might also decide to change careers completely—and find that you excel at something you never imagined. Whatever you do to retain your comfortable level of productivity, your loved ones should respect and support you in it. Also, you should applaud the accomplishments of others, even if you feel a twinge of jealousy that they are able to do things that you can no longer strive to do.

Of course, if you are in a relationship that does not fit into the mold, that does not mean that you cut it off. All relationships, whether they be between friends, family, spouses, or coworkers, take time and work. Patiently try to work out the rough spots with friendships that you treasure. You might find you achieve a higher level of respect, understanding, and love.

TIP: Once Again, Practice Saying No

A useful skill to hone early on is that of defining boundaries. Because there will be times when others will want you to participate in activities you are not up to, you will need to become comfortable with saying no. Understand that you are not failing as a friend, a parent, or an employee when you have to cancel plans or bow out of doing something that everyone wants you to do. Try to explain to those involved that you sometimes have certain limitations, and that this is one of those times. Know that there will be people who will never understand, who might even turn away from you because of your illness. But appreciate those who stand by you, who accept you, lupus and all. They are the people who will, ultimately, make up the core of support and comfort in your life.

Communication Is Key

Throughout your battle with lupus, communication is one of the most important skills to practice. You need to communicate clearly with your physician and the other medical professionals who treat you. And you need to communicate with your loved ones.

When you are first diagnosed, and if it is feasible, invite your loved ones to meet with you and your doctor. Tell them they should feel free to ask whatever questions they have; assure them that no question is stupid, and that your physician is more than willing to explain the disease and its ramifications to them.

Share written material about lupus with your family members

and encourage them to do research on their own. With more eyes looking for information, more valuable and helpful data may come to light.

Lupus is a difficult disease for many people to understand, especially if they have not been exposed to it before. You will need to patiently but firmly communicate your symptoms and the way lupus affects you, and you might find you have to repeat yourself several times before your loved ones comprehend what the disease does to your life. For example, if you have small children and need your parents to help take care of them when you are in a flare, you might need to explain the nature of your fatigue, which is very different from that which your mother and father experienced when they had small children. Patiently explain that a "catnap" won't take care of the bone-numbing fatigue you feel; you need much more rest than that.

Even when you are not in a flare, you need to be under a doctor's care and take appropriate precautions. Your family, however, might be so relieved to see you feeling better that they might press you to get back to normal. They might even believe that you are cured.

In as loving a way as possible, explain to your family that lupus is chronic and that you still need to be mindful of things such as becoming overtired, exposing yourself to too much sun, and coming into contact with infection.

Family

Those closest to you might have the toughest time coping with your disease. It could be terrifying for them to come to terms with your illness, and it could be difficult for you to see them carry on in relatively good health while you struggle.

As you experience more of the physical limitations of lupus, and the financial and practical challenges that arise from it, your family could share the stress of helping you cope. They are, naturally, the people you would turn to for help taking care of your children, doing chores, being available when unexpected complications arise, providing financial assistance when medical costs soar. But these things can strain the best of families, and you might find your relationships with parents and siblings, even extended family members, unraveling at a time when you need them most.

Accepting a Helping Hand

Your family members will undoubtedly want to help you as you face the challenges of lupus. Sometimes their help will be welcome, but sometimes it will feel overwhelming, possibly even smothering.

Your need to maintain some level of independence will change as your disease ebbs and flows. Still, there will be times when your energy and/or physical limitations preclude your being completely able to take care of yourself. At these times, when your family members approach you about doing something to help, try to welcome their intentions warmly, even if you feel irritated; it is the best way they know how to reach out to you in your time of need.

Sometimes, however, you might feel like your family is interfering with your life beyond simply helping you get through flares. Then, tell them that you appreciate their efforts but need to have some degree of autonomy, especially when you are feeling better. Promise them that you will tell them when you need help, and then follow through by giving them the opportunity to assist you in something that you truly do need help with.

Spouses

"For better, for worse. In sickness and in health."

In the heady, exciting throes of a marriage ceremony, many people do not seriously think about the downside of their vows. A wedding is a time of joy, and hopes for the future center only around the benefits of uniting with someone you love. But the marriage vows also allow for times when life is not altogether smooth: ". . . for worse. In sickness . . ." And, as you have found out, those times can come to even the strongest of couples.

Lupus *is* the "worse." It *is* the "sickness." It can bring unexpected financial, time, and personal constraints to a marriage, particularly if there are children involved, too. And because it is chronic, it will be a factor in your marriage from the day of diagnosis forward. Some spouses are able to accept that and adapt to the marriage accordingly. Others find that they are incapable of living with a sick spouse.

Give and Take

Communication from the very beginning is crucial to keeping relationships alive in a marriage where one partner has lupus. This means not only communicating about the disease, but also keeping intact the daily flow of feelings, ideas, and events that make up any marriage. It includes not only talking, but relating in affectionate and intimate ways.

Having a chronic disease can take over almost all your waking (and sleeping) moments. But sometimes you will have to set aside your concerns about the disease and focus on your spouse's concerns. Stay interested in your spouse's life and try not to let the lupus distance you from him or her. Of course, sometimes you will have to lovingly and patiently insist that you need to take care of yourself rather than stay up late, engage in an energetic activity, or take time to be available to your spouse. But having lupus does not mean that you "check out" of your spouse's life entirely.

With lupus in the picture, you and your spouse will need to work harder at being a couple, respecting each other and encouraging your love to strengthen in the face of the health challenge that has come into the marriage. If you have severe joint pain, you will need to experiment with new positions and activities that will continue to promote intimacy between you. If you become unable to work, you should develop a financial plan that will take in your spouse's needs as well as your own. And if you have children, you still need to be active in their upbringing, providing moral support to your spouse when you cannot physically take on certain parenting duties.

When a Marriage Ends

The benefits of staying with your spouse and achieving a new, higher level of love and respect can outweigh the pain and hard work of getting there. However, some marriages are fragile to begin with, or were entered into for less than loving reasons. In these cases, sometimes the spouses cannot work out their differences in the face of a chronic illness. The ensuing divorce can be a time of great anguish for the lupus patient, especially if he or she is in the throes of a flare.

Remember to take care of yourself, body and soul, if you find yourself going through a divorce. Rely on your friends and family to provide you with moral, financial, and physical support. Pray and meditate to ease your stress, and focus on the time when the trauma of breaking up your marriage will be behind you, and you can get on with your life, building it up to something better than before.

Children

Being a parent is one of the truly wonderful gifts of life, and children are a source of great joy and happiness. However, with lupus in the mix, being a parent becomes more challenging and painful.

The most obvious factor that inhibits your ability to be a fully present parent is your lack of energy. You might not have the ability to chase a toddler (or two!) around the house all day, and you might not be able to chauffeur older children to and from their after-school activities.

A close network of friends and fellow parents can help ease your burden. Being part of a carpool can save you the burden of driving every day, and shopping with other mothers can make it easier to take care of your errands *and* small children.

Even if you cannot afford full-time child care, seek ways that you can get a qualified individual to watch your child or children so that you can at least get a nap in the afternoon. A church community can also be a source of help, especially for those times when a flare unexpectedly intrudes upon your daily activities.

As your children get older, enlist their help in running the household. This does not mean that you hand over the keys to the kingdom, but it does mean that you give them specific, doable chores that they are expected to carry out on a regular basis. This can not only relieve you of some of the burden of daily work, but it can also teach your children valuable lessons in responsibility and reaching out to help when someone is ill.

Lupus from a Child's Perspective

Even if they are extremely bright, young children have a limited emotional capacity to understand that Mommy or Daddy can be ill even though she or he looks healthy. They might become so fearful as to believe their parent will die, and this insecurity could lead to their acting out with inappropriate behavior.

Because lupus is a difficult disease for adults to understand, do not assume that your explanation will be comprehended by your young child. Going into a lengthy explanation of lupus and the nature of flares could backfire and bring about more confusion than clarity. Address instead the relationship you have with your child, and the continuity of your love for him or her. Reassure your child that Mommy's or Daddy's illness is not life threatening, and that he or she will feel better soon. Emphasize the constancy of the lupus parent's presence in the child's life, and encourage your child to communicate his or her fears openly.

A child psychologist can work with the lupus patient's doctor to set up an effective way to handle a youngster's fears if these become overwhelming. Other family members can help, too, by treating the lupus patient with as much steadiness and normalcy as possible. It does a young child no good to see adults becoming emotionally distraught over the health condition of his or her parent.

Older children also might find it difficult to accept a parent who is limited by a chronic illness. Their feelings could center around fear, but they will also probably be tinged with anger that Mom or Dad is not available to them and cannot take them places or do things with them. Especially with teenagers, this is a perfect opportunity to teach an important lesson about becoming aware of the needs of others.

Reassure your older child that you love and treasure him or her, but also reinforce your need to tend to your health. Ask your child to help you (not to take on the bulk of your care, but to help in some smaller way). Engage in activities with your child when you feel up to it.

Friends

Having friends with whom you can share the good and bad times is extremely important. Having lupus can in some ways be a blessing in disguise; through your illness you will discover who is a true friend and who is a fair-weather friend. In other words, those people who truly care about you will stand with you through lupus. Those people who are more superficial, who are less accepting of the challenges of being human, will fall away.

Remember to Be a Friend, Too

Having a chronic illness is a very attention- and time-consuming occupation. When you engage in relationships with other people, however, you must remember to be interested in them, to reach out to them and address their needs and fears, too. Take care of yourself, of course. But do not let your world revolve solely around yourself. Otherwise you will find your circle of friends dwindling rapidly.

The Fluidity of Friendship

How many of us had a best friend when we were little? And how many of us have maintained that fast friendship through to adulthood?

Friendships can be forever, but they can be fluid, too, ebbing and flowing with who we are and what we do at any particular time in our lives. Geography plays a part in making and maintaining friendships, as does a variety of other issues, such as marriage and/or parenting status, occupation, and religious beliefs. We would like to believe that the friends we have today will be the friends we have tomorrow. But sometimes, even without lupus, that is just not possible.

As you tell your friends about your disease, you will notice a range of reactions, from sympathy to disbelief to distancing. Try not to take the reactions too personally; you are not responsible for the emotional reactions of others.

Sometimes people are not emotionally ready to deal with the chronic illness of another. If that is the case with one or more of your friends, you will feel pain and loss. But realize that you must respect your friend or friends for who they are. Do what you have to do, and let them have the same freedom.

It is natural to mourn any friendships that fall apart because of lupus. However, you should rejoice in the friendships that remain and become stronger in spite of the disease. Also, having lupus will expose you to a whole population of incredible, strong people who are also coping with the disease. These people will become friends and, in many cases, become an even more wonderful presence in your life than any friends before.

Dating for the Lupus Patient

If you are not married or in a relationship when you are diagnosed, there is no need to believe that your dating life is over. In some ways, having lupus while dating can help you quickly discern which potential partners are able to cope with adversity and which are not. You can find out a great deal about a person's capacity for empathy and his or her willingness to help others. You can potentially find yourself in a more nurturing, uplifting, loving relationship than you ever felt possible.

But you have to jump into the dating pond before you can get to that point!

Sorting through the Possibilities

The ways in which lupus patients go about finding people to date are very much the same as those of the general population. Personal referrals, chance meetings, dating services, church singles groups— all these hold potential for finding new friends and, possibly, love interests.

"The more you fill your life with things that interest you, the more you bring interesting people into your life," says Carolyn Dodge, vice president of Patient and Community Services with the Arthritis Foundation. "When you start to get excited about your own life, that's when you meet people like yourself, friends who can introduce you to that special person."

First Impressions

When you meet someone for the first time, try not to wear your lupus on your sleeve. Gauge how much you want to trust the person you are with, and give him or her information appropriately.

"Most men I meet, I tell straightaway," says Dodge, who has suffered from rheumatoid arthritis since childhood and works with arthritis and lupus patients in workshops on dating. "I don't go into a huge dissertation of what that entails, but bring it up just to let them know. It's a wonderful way to weed out the goonies! Because I have arthritis, it helps me weed out those who don't have empathy and who can't deal with some of the bigger issues. I haven't spent a lot of time with those who don't have empathy."

Still, you do not have to feel obligated to mention lupus on the first date. If you are comfortable mentioning it, fine. But if you sense that the other person might not be empathic, or appears to want something from the relationship that you cannot give, feel free to back off.

Of course, if the person you are meeting suggests you sit in an outdoor café under the blazing sun, or wants you to accompany him or her on a hike up a mountain when you suffer from joint pain, you will need to set limits. Explain that your medical condition prevents you from enjoying these activities, and gauge the other person's reaction. But do not feel obligated to go into great detail. You will need to share lupus with the person you allow closely into your life, but you do not need to share it with everyone.

Sex and Lupus

In Victorian times, and even as recently as fifty years ago, sexual encounters did not put too much emphasis on male performance in bed and did not require women from that time to have an unappeasable appetite for making love. In today's celluloid and prose, men are often portrayed as Greek Adonises with an unlimited ability to make love, and women are portrayed to be always ready and willing and have well-endowed bodies. If one adds the pressure of living with a painful and chronic condition such as lupus to the sexual expectations that men and women have to live up to in a relationship, it is not surprising that more than 50 percent of marriages in which one of the partners has lupus ends in divorce.

Problems with sexual activity in lupus patients are due to generalized symptoms, coexisting conditions, or specific problems with the sexual organs. Generalized symptoms that interfere with sexual activity include painful and stiff joints that limit mobility of the hips, upper body, or spine due to active disease or due to side effects from prolonged use of steroids. The use of this medication can also cause excessive fat accumulation in the face, neck, and stomach, which may be unsightly to one's partner and may cause a severe loss of self-esteem in the lupus patient that also affects the person's sexual performance. Unpredictable, severe mental and physical fatigue can prevent the person from engaging in passionate pursuits.

Depression is altogether too common in lupus patients due to the effects on the brain from this illness, and this can decrease one's libido or desire for sexual activity. Other diseases that coexist with lupus that can impede the ability to have sexual intercourse include high blood pressure and diabetes, which can decrease the blood circulation to sex organs. Many of the medications used to treat these conditions may cause delay in ejaculation, delayed or absent orgasms, and an inability to have or sustain erections. Although depression decreases one's libido, the medications used to treat the condition may also cause these side effects.

Premature menopause may result from the use of chemotherapy in older women. This may result in lack of lubrication of the sexual organs and also in some thinning and fragility of the vaginal lining. Not all lupus patients are candidates for hormone replacement, especially if they have antibodies that predispose them to blood clots in their veins. Sjögren's syndrome, which causes dry eyes and dry mouth, also causes dryness of the vagina due to the immune attack on the glands, and exists with lupus in about 20 percent of patients. When fibromyalgia exists with lupus, then problems such as vulvodynia, which is pain when penetration is attempted, may be present. Changing positions can help alleviate pressure on the area that causes pain on entry.

If a lupus patient has an understanding and supportive partner, most of the above problems can be worked out by minimizing the duration of medications that cause side effects, taking warm baths to relieve stiffness and joint pain, and use of lubricants if needed. Communication between the partners and with their health-care provider is key to solving these issues.

Is He or She "the One"?

"A lot of times," says Dodge, "people will become more sexually available when they've been diagnosed with a chronic illness. This is because it gives them validation, but that's really the wrong reason. You should never put yourself in an intimate situation until you come to love and trust your partner for who he or she is. Take time to figure out who you're looking for. Don't settle for someone because you think, 'That's all there is.'"

Time is a very important element in finding out who someone is. So is experiencing a number of things together. If you have lupus and are dating someone, one hopes you will have a good idea of how your relationship fares through flares and times of better health. Still, sometimes there are aspects of a relationship that do not come up until a couple is married. And these can be particularly serious points when one of the partners has lupus.

- **Children.** Many women who have lupus can have children; however, there are certain considerations that a couple contemplating children should take into account. For example, the spouse without lupus must understand that there could be times when he or she will be the sole parent, while his or her partner is suffering from a flare. The "healthy" spouse should be able to take on these tasks with willingness and commitment.
- **Finances.** A person who has lupus might have to cut back on working, or stop working altogether. The "healthy" partner should understand this and be willing to reevaluate his or her lifestyle needs in order to accommodate the health needs of his or her spouse.
- **Physical Constraints.** Lupus can alter a person's psyche and physique. The "healthy" partner should find joy in his or her relationship without putting too heavy an emphasis on the lupus patient's looks. And he or she should be ready and able to provide moral support when times are hard and the lupus patient is particularly fragile.
- **Lifestyle Considerations.** In any successful relationship, there is a spirit of compromise. However, when one partner has lupus, sometimes compromise is not possible. For example, if the "healthy" spouse is offered a job opportunity in another city, no matter how attractive that offer might be, it

may not be feasible because of the health condition of his or her spouse. Likewise, there might be times when attending family functions is impossible, or travel plans must be changed, due to lupus flares or complications. The healthy spouse needs to be extremely flexible and willing to give a bit more than in a relationship where both partners are healthy.

Planning a Life Together

With lupus, it is almost impossible to plan and be assured that your plans will remain intact. But life can bring change even when lupus is not in the picture. Marriage vows allow for good times *and* bad times. The successful couple will realize that life holds no guarantees—the way to happiness together is through commitment to each other, to the marriage vows, and to a sense of love and laughter that keeps you together through it all.

Letting Go of People

When you are first diagnosed with lupus, one of your impulses might be to cling to everything and everyone in your life "before." You might find yourself assuring your friends that nothing has changed, and you might even engage in activities that are detrimental to your new state of health because you don't want to let go of certain relationships. For example, if all your friends used to go to the beach, you might still accompany them even though you know you shouldn't be out in the sun.

Although this reaction is natural, it can hold you back from optimizing your health and learning how to best cope with your life with lupus. It can bring on more undue stress. It might even cause you worse physical trouble and lead to a dangerous progression of the disease.

As you work through your emotions regarding lupus, try to maintain objectivity about your relationships. Be realistic about their depth and the honesty on which they are based. Understand that your life has changed, and of necessity your friends will need to understand that, too, or you will have to move on.

Moving on means accepting people as they are, and accepting yourself as you are. It means not harboring resentment for what you perceive to be someone else's failings. Rather, it means being aware of your needs and the needs of others. It means accepting when the

How Can a Woman with Lupus Best Prepare Herself to Have Children?

Ninety percent of patients with lupus are women, and three-quarters of these women are in their teenage or childbearing years. It is possible for young women with lupus to even go through chemotherapy for organ-threatening lupus and preserve fertility and have babies.

However, lupus can cause complications during pregnancy when it is active or when phospholipid antibodies or anti-Ro antibodies are present. It is best for women with lupus to get pregnant when their doctors tell them that their illness is not active. If that is the case but the above antibodies are present, an aspirin a day may prevent miscarriages due to antiphospholipid antibodies, and careful monitoring with fetal cardiac ultrasound will be necessary to detect fetal cardiac problems due to the anti-Ro antibody.

About a third of lupus patients have a flare-up of lupus during pregnancy, particularly if their disease was active at the outset.

Many of the medications used to treat lupus cannot be used during pregnancy because of possible toxic effects on the developing fetus. Some medications, such as methotrexate, must be stopped a few menstrual cycles prior to getting pregnant, and others, such as hydroxychloroquine, can be continued till pregnancy is diagnosed.

Chemotherapy for kidney involvement from lupus can cause ovarian failure or testicular failure and subsequent infertility. The older the woman and the higher the cumulative dose of chemotherapy, the higher her chance of infertility. Avoiding chemotherapy for aggressive kidney disease may result in kidney failure, which absolutely rules out conception and a successful pregnancy. Sperm donation, storage of fertilized eggs, and suppressing ovulation during chemotherapy can help circumvent the problem.

change in your life encourages you to move into more nurturing, uplifting friendships and away from less adaptable ones.

Determining when to move away from someone and how to communicate it is not easy. Rely on your inner voice, the place of peace that you find in your prayer or meditation, to guide you through the transition. And know that all is not lost—you will find strong relationships among those you already have and those to come if you only believe.

16

THE RELATIONSHIP FACTOR:

Especially for People Whose Loved Ones Have Lupus

Nothing can be more upsetting than seeing someone you love struggle with a disease, especially one that is chronic and for which there is no cure. As a spouse, parent, sibling, or friend, you want to feel helpful; you want to take away the pain. But where lupus is involved, this might seem impossible.

Although you cannot offer medicinal cures for your loved one's pain, there are things that you can do to maintain your relationship and bring comfort to your loved one with lupus. Some of these things are tangible and directly impact the lupus patient. Other things are more internal in nature, and help you cope. All of these things and more will help keep you close to the person you care about and make you both feel better.

The Most Common Stress Factors

No relationship is stress-free. However, when lupus enters the picture, stress points that existed before can be magnified, and new stresses can emerge. Some of the most common stress factors in a lupus-influenced relationship stem from:

• **Financial Concerns.** Lupus can be a very expensive illness. If you live with a loved one with lupus, it is essential that you both take stock of your financial situation and work together to adapt to the new parameters of your lives with lupus. Don't let the financial issues get between you and your loved one.

- **Lifestyle Changes.** Sometimes your loved one is able to function almost normally, and sometimes he or she is bedridden. Besides experiencing a distancing between you and your loved one when the pain and other symptoms take hold, your own group of friends and family might become more remote. You need to work with your loved one to keep communication and relationships going.
- **Intimacy.** On a very personal level, the intimacy you enjoyed between you and your loved one may also change because of lupus. The pain your loved one experiences, and the emotional burden of dealing with a chronic disease, can change the landscape of the physical ways you relate to one another. You might even begin to think you are no longer "in love" with the person you married, the person who now seems closer to lupus than to you.
- **Children.** Being a parent is hard work, but being a parent with a spouse who has lupus compounds the difficulty many times over. There will be times when your spouse cannot be Mommy or Daddy, but must be a patient, and you must carry the responsibility for the household. At times you will feel as though you are responsible for the whole world—and you might feel yourself caving under that pressure.

Help for Your Extra Stress

As your life changes in ways you could not imagine before lupus, you need to take personal time to reflect, meditate, and/or pray to firmly establish priorities that will enable you to cope. Through this introspection you may find that discovering the joy of relationships without pressure to mold them to specific activities or schedules will release some of the pressure of the unpredictability of lupus.

Never forget that you might need help at times, too—and don't be afraid to reach out for it. Whether in the form of counseling, support groups, or reliance upon family and friends, you need to take care of yourself in order to take care of others. Also, remember that lupus is a chronic disease and will be part of the landscape of your life for a very long time. Continue seeing to your own physical, emotional, and spiritual health in between flares, and keep looking for new ways to better enjoy your family life in spite of lupus.

Finding alternatives to usual activities is another way to ease your and your loved one's stress level. For example, if your loved one is too ill to go out, developing hobbies or leisure activities together that are compatible with staying closer to home can maintain your own level of activity while adapting to the constraints of your loved one's disease.

Coping with Changes in Intimacy

Finding ways to cope with the changes in the intimacy of your relationship should not be ignored. Try to discover new ways of relating, looking upon this process of discovery as an adventure, rather than a duty. Be aware of the myriad of ways you can bring comfort to one another and express your affection in spite of lupus. Consult with your loved one's physician and see if there might be physical reasons for some of your problems. For example, vaginal dryness may be due to autoimmune destruction of lubricating glands or due to estrogen deficiency. A decreased libido and an inability to sustain erections may be due to depression, side effects of medications, or decreased blood flow. Your loved one's physician can work with you to find tangible solutions to these and other problems. And, if need be, seeking further help via counseling can make your relationship stronger, too.

Indeed, it is important to communicate your needs and work together to find ways to adapt. Ignoring the disease and its effect on your lives, or doing too many activities on your own may result in a deep rift between you and your loved one that cannot be bridged.

Lupus through the Eyes of Those Who Care

If you are committed to a relationship with a loved one who has lupus, identifying the stresses that buffet both of you can help tremendously in coping with the disease. Equally important is knowing that you are not alone in your struggle. You can learn a great deal from those who are in similar situations, and help them, too, as they cope with lupus in their lives. Here is what some caring others have to say:

"Once somebody has a chronic illness, things will never be normal again," says Jason, who has been married to Sylvia for eighteen years.

"Before she was diagnosed with lupus, I didn't have any strong feelings about her physical health," says Ann, the mother of Desiree. "The diagnosis was a shock, and afterward there was a complete upheaval in my own thinking about her well-being."

"Prior to her diagnosis, it was very confusing. I knew something was wrong, but the problem with lupus is that you don't look sick necessarily," says Phil, who has been married to Patty for twenty-one years. "After her diagnosis, I still didn't know what lupus was. But we've both been learning a lot."

"With any chronic disease, there's an element of surprise," says Doug, who has been married to Becky for almost seventeen years. "With lupus, you're bound to have surprises; you just never know what each day will bring."

Surprise, disbelief, not knowing what lupus is or what it means—these are a few of the reactions of loved ones at the onset of the lupus diagnosis. And they are all perfectly natural.

Larry, cofacilitator of a lupus support group for caring others, says, "It's okay to be angry, okay to have regrets, to vent. As long as you have the perspective that you ultimately will have to understand that your life and their life will change."

While you grapple with these internal emotions, which are often powerful and painful, the lupus patient is trying to understand what the diagnosis means and struggling with physical symptoms that are often painful and frightening.

In the first weeks and months following diagnosis, there can be much misunderstanding and inadvertent hurt inflicted on one or both people. Harsh words can be spoken out of frustration at the situation, anger at the disease, or fear of the future. A lupus patient taking prednisone may be prone to sharp mood swings that make life stormy. The loved one may feel pressure to be strong at a time when he or she feels weakest. The financial burden associated with medical care and lost wages may take a toll. As pressures increase, so do misunderstandings. Your relationship begins to unravel at a time when it needs to be strongest.

The most important thing you can do for your loved one now is to learn as much as you can about the disease and communicate your desire to be supportive. Physical closeness is important, but so is the reassurance that you are willing to listen and help in any way needed. And, of course, following through on that promise is vital as well.

"Don't try to hide the fact that the person has lupus," says Larry. "If people on the outside make wisecracks, you can just ignore it or gently give them some information. That helps a lot."

Communicating your own thoughts and concerns about the changes lupus brings is important, too. So is everyday communication, talking about the big and little things that make up a relationship beyond lupus.

"You have to keep the flow of information going," says Phil. "If she doesn't speak up, if you don't speak up, that's a problem."

It is also important not to be judgmental. Your loved one did not ask to be given lupus, nor does he or she know how lupus developed. You can be assured that he or she already asked, "I wonder when I did this to myself?" over and over and came up with no answer, because there is none. Putting the blame on an event or person is counterproductive to facing the bald fact: Your loved one has lupus, and you both have to move forward from there.

Lupus and the Family: The Physician's Role

Many aspects of lupus can interfere with day-to-day activities with one's loved ones. Children find it difficult that their parent has to spend time resting instead of playing with them, and important outdoor events for them have to be planned carefully in order to avoid excessive sun exposure for their parent. Spouses may come home to find that their loved one has gone to bed because they have no energy to stay up with them. Patients can become despondent because of their illness or from side effects of their medications, and this can take a toll on the relationship between couples.

A visit that is scheduled with your doctor to discuss issues that have come up in the family is often helpful. Inform your doctor ahead of time that you are making this visit with your spouse or children to answer some questions about your illness.

A Helping Hand

One of the best ways to show support and gain a better understanding of your loved one's situation is to ask his or her primary-care physician for a conference appointment. No physical exam will take place. Rather, in a calm setting away from home, you, the patient, and the doctor can talk about the specific implications of the disease, address questions, and discuss a course of action that will help smooth the way for the transition into a life with lupus. Again, try not to be judgmental when it comes to your loved one's selection of a physician. Each person has different likes and dislikes, and you must respect your loved one's right to choose his or her own doctor.

After the initial meeting, follow-up conferences might also be needed as time and the disease's course unfolds. The physician may suggest counseling, either individual or joint, where issues can be grappled with at greater length. Some people are not comfortable with counseling, but it can help tremendously to clear away misunderstandings and further the focus on issues and solutions. Be open-minded and flexible. Life with lupus demands flexibility.

Get Support

Support groups promote a sense of community, a network of others who have gone through many similar situations and who have ideas about how to handle them, based on their own experience. There are support groups for patients and some for caring others, where loved ones can share their thoughts, struggles, and suggestions with one another.

"I went through the transition from denial to having a fatalistic outlook, to acceptance and participation," says Larry, husband of a lupus patient. "Then I really started thinking, 'I'm not out here by myself with these thoughts and feelings of frustration. I'm sure a lot of people are dealing with these problems.' When you disconnect emotionally, you pay for it down the road."

While some support groups can degenerate into gripe sessions, the best ones are those that strive to be productive. You and your loved one might need to shop around before finding one that you like, but your search will be worth the time.

Throughout the United States, the Lupus Foundation of America's local chapters sponsor support groups for patients and caring others. In addition, the Arthritis Foundation and local hospitals often sponsor such groups and other forums devoted to patient support. Your doctor is an excellent source of information for contacting these organizations in your area. In addition, a list of national resources can be found in the back of this book.

Avoid Taking Control

In the first days and months after diagnosis, the lupus patient is discovering the ways in which his or her lupus is manifesting itself. During this time, you might have a tendency to take over complete control, to hover over your loved one and think you are helping. Actually, this can have the opposite effect.

"I come from a family where men usually fix things," says John. "In the beginning, I found myself wanting to do more, to do something, to make things better, to be the warrior."

Knowing when to step in requires observation, understanding, and a willingness to communicate. It *can* be done.

John says, "When she will allow it, I will do any and all tasks, from laundry to shopping to purchasing her new automobile. But I'm always careful to ask, 'May I?' or 'Would you mind if . . . ?' so she never feels as though she can't. I don't want to take any of that away from her."

The mother of a lupus patient agrees. "Smothering can be carried to extremes," says Ann. "Once the person has been diagnosed and he or she knows what it entails, there's a lot they have to do themselves. But it is extremely important to be a good listener and help if it is wanted."

Of course, if you see your loved one doing something detrimental to his or her health, such as going off medication without a doctor's supervision or ignoring serious symptoms, you might need to step in more firmly. But otherwise, try to respect boundaries that will allow your loved one to still feel productive, even in the face of chronic illness.

Be Flexible

Being in a relationship with a lupus patient requires flexibility, especially when it comes to scheduling activities. You might be ready to leave for dinner and your loved one will suddenly say he or she is just too tired. Or you might plan a trip together, only to have it fall apart because of a flare. In those cases, it is important to keep in mind priorities: what is important, and what is expendable.

"Lupus doesn't rule my life," says John. "It bends things. We might miss the Friday-night movie, but that doesn't mean we'll miss the Saturday movie. Or we may not be able to eat out five times a week. But those are superficial things. All the things you bend to are all superficial."

"There are some days she's just done-in because of lupus, and she can't function," says Phil. "So I can offer options and let her decide. I'm there to advise, suggest, and be the listening board. That's a big help."

Doug says, "It's important to treat your sick spouse or girlfriend with as much normalcy as possible. And you have to keep a sense of humor about it."

Anticipating circumstances can help ease your loved one's pain. For example, parking near your destination will make it easier on the lupus patient. Scheduling activities around your loved one's rest periods will also be essential—and much appreciated!

If you spend a great deal of time with a lupus patient, it is helpful to have basic information available to you. For example, you should know whom to contact in case of emergency and the name of the lupus patient's medical insurance, and have a sense of allergies and medications that he or she is taking. It may be helpful for you to know CPR and basic first aid; however, any other intervention measures are best left to medical professionals.

Taking Care of Yourself

If you are not careful, lupus can weigh heavily on your mind, time, and other resources, causing increased stress and possibly exacerbating your own health problems. If this happens, it will be more difficult to extend assistance to your loved one. It is essential to take care of yourself and find appropriate activities that can help you minimize your stress and anxiety.

"I always have activities outside the home, especially classic-car restoration," says Larry. "I'm really now starting to enjoy and value family life, too. For instance, I can play on the computer at home."

Javier, who cofacilitates the caring-others support group with Larry, says, "I take personal time. I belong to a bowling league, and I'll also work on the computer at home. That way we have time to ourselves, but we're there for each other, too."

Another area that needs to be addressed is the health of the caregiver. When the focus is so frequently on the lupus patient's health, sometimes the supportive spouse, parent, or sibling overlooks his or her own health concerns, physical and emotional.

"When I have a cold," says Clara, daughter of Aura, "I sometimes feel bad to be complaining at all, because it can't be nearly as bad as how my mother feels. But you have to take time out for yourself, as well."

"I think I'm expected to be strong, not have the emotions, cry, or express worries or concerns," says Chrissie, who has cared about and for Mary for ten years. "What I've done is have my own private times with these stresses."

Develop Spiritually

For your sake, as well as your loved one's, you must keep up with your own emotional and medical status and maintain a healthy diet and exercise regimen. You should do all that is necessary to take care of your condition if you do fall ill, and rely on your loved one for support and help as much as possible.

If you care about someone with lupus, you can benefit also from a strong spiritual life when changes shake up your relationship and the well-being of your loved one. In some studies, even remote prayer can bring benefits to someone who suffers, so you need not even be present with your loved one to bring him or her some solace through supplication.

"It took a couple of years to calm down," says Chrissie. "Now I kind of renewed my spiritual side and pray a lot. There's been more optimism within me."

How you pray for your loved one will be determined by what method you are usually comfortable with. However, try to pray constructively, asking for guidance, peace, and comfort, rather than using an all-or-nothing approach (asking for a complete cure and nothing else). This way, you will be asking for immediate healing and, one hopes, be bringing a sense of calm to the situation. Asking for a complete cure instead can bring on feelings of frustration and disappointment that God sees your loved one as unworthy of a total cure.

Any relationship will have its highs and lows, but with lupus in the picture, the relationship can be even more charged with difficulties. Keeping your own sense of self and peace will help you

> ## TIP: Encourage Your Loved One
>
> The lupus patient can assist his or her caregivers, too, in reducing the stress of living with a chronic illness. You should feel free to encourage your loved one to find his or her strengths and discover victories within the struggle against lupus.

cope, and give even more reassurance to your loved one that you will continue to support him or her through it all.

Looking Ahead

Looking ahead and setting (or resetting) priorities will also help you adjust to your and your loved one's new life.

"My priority is always Meg," says John. "For those caregivers who find that the job within their profession doesn't meet their personal goals, make a change so that you can work in an environment that allows you the physical and emotional freedom to do what you have to do for your mate or spouse."

"You have to be practical. You can't dwell on what might have been if your child, spouse, or loved one didn't have lupus. You have to love that person through everything," says Ann. "There's no alternative, unless you sever yourself from the relationship."

Letting Go

Sad to say, sometimes lupus exacts such a toll on husbands and wives, parents and children, friends and coworkers that relationships split apart.

From his experience as cofacilitator of a support group for caring others, Larry says, "Those who tend to cope best are those who are in a very loving, give-and-take type of relationship. If the relationship is too one-sided, there seems to be a lot less capability there to cope. Some families just fall apart. Some families don't realize what's going on and they refuse to accept it. There are different stages that you go through. One of them is denial. And that can go on forever."

Javier, who works with Larry as cofacilitator of the support group, agrees. "Denial is insidious to the relationship. With lupus, there are long-term consequences. People don't want to look at it like that. They want to think it's going to be short-term, that the patient is going to get over it down the road. After months, years, people get frustrated."

Drawing people out of denial is one of the things Javier tries to do in the support group. "I use the elephant analogy. It's big, but you can eat one if you take it one bite at a time. You can take the same approach with lupus."

Still, many relationships fall apart because of lupus.

"People will do one of two things," says Javier. "Either they will work it out together and work out their hopes and dreams together, or they won't do well with it. They become self-focused. But with people who have a strong relationship anyway, lupus will make them stronger."

Moving Forward

Before you sever a relationship with a loved one who has lupus, examine the reasons you are breaking away. Think of the times you have shared, the affection between you, and the promises you have made. Ask yourself tough questions about your reasons for being in the relationship before lupus. Were they selfish reasons? Or has there truly been a mutual, meaningful relationship between you and the lupus patient? And now that lupus is a factor, ask yourself what has changed, what you are willing to do, and what you are willing to give.

Perhaps you will see that your relationship was not strong to begin with. Perhaps you will discover that your reasons for being together were more mercenary than mutual.

But perhaps, by looking carefully at all the aspects of the relationship, you will find that there isn't a drastic change in your affection, just a change in the externals of it. Your desire to be part of your loved one's life may actually be strengthened by the challenges lupus brings, and your realization of the support you have for one another may increase as you see that your loved one wants to reach out to you, too, in spite of lupus.

"It all depends on how much you love somebody," says Doug. "If you love somebody, you will give it your best shot."

Amid the trials, there are many pleasant discoveries awaiting you as you care for a "lupie." Your extra efforts to support your loved one can be beneficial to both of you.

Phil says, "I'm part of her and she's part of me. We're part of each other. There is comfort in that."

The Genetic Connection

A question that often comes up in young couples who have newly wed is whether their child will have a high risk of getting lupus.

Though genes influence the development of lupus, even pairs of identical twins who have exactly the same copies of genes are not always concordant for lupus. In other words, only 50 percent of twin siblings with an identical twin with lupus will get lupus during their lifetime. In more common circumstances, such as one parent with lupus, the risk is much less and is estimated to be around 1 percent. Since autoimmune illnesses such as lupus, thyroid disease, psoriasis, and skin depigmentation often cluster in families, the risk of any autoimmune diseases in children of a parent with lupus is about 15 percent.

17

THE RELATIONSHIP FACTOR:

The Lupus Community

Being diagnosed with lupus need not be the end of a happy life. Rather, it can be the beginning of new, nurturing relationships and fulfilling experiences. You will be challenged, of course, and your life will go through major changes. But on the positive side, you will get to know yourself better than ever before, and in so doing you will come to a greater respect for the courage and strength you possess in the face of a difficult and painful situation. And you will open new horizons on many levels: personal, productive, and spiritual.

The Lupus Community

The men and women who comprise the lupus community are an impressive group of people. Rheumatologists must be extremely patient and perceptive to unravel extremely complex sets of symptoms and treatments. They must have the personal skills to communicate intricate concepts and courses of treatment to people who are, naturally, worried and confused over what is happening to their bodies. And, perhaps most important, they must have patience and resolve to continue to treat patients whose chronic illnesses mean that, by default, they are not curable.

The pharmacists, nurses, and other medical professionals who assist rheumatologists and their patients must also be highly skilled and intuitive. Support organizations and their personnel must be ever ready to adapt to the changing needs of their constituents.

But perhaps the most impressive of all the members of the lupus community are the patients themselves. These men, women, and children must withstand tremendous pain, setbacks, health surprises, and spiritual assaults. In order to get beyond the trials to achieve a good quality of life, they must have tenacious perseverance and innate hope. They must develop deep reserves of self-motivation. And they must also know when to ask for help.

Where to Turn for Support

Even if you have always been an independent person who thrives on personal achievement, once you are diagnosed with lupus, you will need physical, emotional, and spiritual support.

The first place to turn to for support is, obviously, your family and friends. However, as you know, sometimes these people might not be able to lend you the immediate support and guidance you need. They might be more confused than you are about what lupus is and what it means to you, or they might fall into denial or other negative emotions regarding your illness.

If you feel you are not being supported appropriately, and if you feel you need more than what your family and friends can offer, you can probably find the support you need within the lupus community's wide network of service organizations.

Lupus Organizations

There are many organizations that serve the lupus community specifically. The Lupus Foundation of America, Inc., is a general umbrella organization for several regional and national groups and initiatives, as well as fund-raising efforts to promote awareness and research. Through their Web site, www.lupus.org, you can access a list of chapters throughout the country, as well as find information about lupus, current events, research programs, and fellow patient support.

The SLE Foundation has a significant presence in New York, and is organizing to broaden its scope to take in other areas. Through it, a number of patient information seminars, fund-raising efforts, and research grants are sponsored. Their Web site, www.lupusny.org, also includes information about the latest lupus-related news and research. Their sister organization, the Lupus Research Institute, gives grants to researchers and tracks lupus studies and their conclusions.

Other regional lupus groups have Web sites that can be accessed by anyone with Internet access. A comprehensive list is available through the Lupus Foundation of America, Inc. As you become more able to cope with your life with lupus, consider volunteering for your local lupus organization, or at the national level. Your contribution is certainly needed and can bring you many benefits, too.

Support Groups and Their Sponsors

Support groups set up by the Arthritis Foundation, the Lupus Foundation, or your local hospital can be a tremendous source of uplifting encouragement and support. Although these groups are not designed to provide psychological counseling or in-depth analysis of an individual's problems, they are usually run by trained facilitators who have extensive experience with lupus and the ramifications of dealing with the disease.

Opening yourself up to a group of people will take a lot of courage and trust on your part. Do not feel you have to dive right in when you first visit a group. See how comfortable you are, and what kind of atmosphere the group generates (is it kind and supportive? complaining and negative?). Be open to trying more than one group at first, so that you can find one that is a good fit with what you need.

It might take you a while to find the support group that is right for you; however, once you do, you will thrive in it. Also, over time you will be amazed at how much your experience can be of assistance to others; the help you get can be given back to other lupus patients who are not quite as far along in their journey as you are.

Related Organizations

Your church or synagogue is another place where you can reach out for help. Having a prayer group focus on your needs can be a very cleansing experience. So, too, can allowing members of the religious community to help you in tangible ways (cooking meals, providing you with transportation to and from doctor appointments, or acting as your advocate if you are hospitalized). These extensions of friendship and faith will be encouraging to you, not to mention stress releasing.

There are also Web sites run by various lupus organizations, as well as general sites that are connected with certain health-related concerns. These sites often offer chat rooms, bulletin boards, and other means by which lupus patients can communicate via the Internet. Although you might be hesitant to speak about your personal health on-line, some patients have found valuable information and guidance through these sources, especially in the days and months following diagnosis.

The Internet can also be a hotbed of false information and dissemination of unfounded stories and urban legends. The Mayo Clinic's Web site, www.mayoclinic.com, offers some tips on how to discern what is fact and what is fiction among the many Web-circulated health stories. Also, a general Web site, www.urbanlegends.about.com, tracks such stories and gives a more balanced take on the information these legends promulgate. Before you become upset or worried over a story you read on the Internet, check with these sources and your doctor to verify the truth of it. And if you have friends who send upsetting information to you frequently, ask them to stop; exposing yourself to such fiction does nothing to help you handle the facts of your life with lupus.

Building Synergies

Lupus has many "cousins"—related diseases and syndromes that share some symptoms and treatments. These include fibromyalgia, Sjögren's syndrome, rheumatoid arthritis, as well as other illnesses. Many of these "lupus cousins" are represented by their own organizations, or have a presence within an umbrella organization (for example, people with rheumatoid arthritis or scleroderma can find information and support through the Arthritis Foundation). These groups can provide you with information about how to deal with shared symptoms and reactions to medications that patients suffering from these ailments might have, too. Some of their programs and seminars are also beneficial to lupus patients, as are some of the research studies that they sponsor, especially where lupus patients also have one or more of these overlap diseases.

Your Attitude toward Support

At first, you might feel hesitant to be a burden on other people, especially those who are strangers to you. But it is precisely for this reason that good-hearted people gather; their commitment to help others in their times of need applies to your situation as much as it does to others in difficult straits. If you do not do so already, learn to trust people's helpfulness and reach out for it gratefully and gracefully.

If you are a highly independent person, allowing others to see you in your weakness might feel awkward or truly terrible to you. Lupus teaches us time and again that we are human—don't be afraid to acknowledge this to yourself and others. Learn to accept the ups and downs, and appreciate the constancy of your support network. It can truly give you much more strength and hope than if you always insist on going it alone.

Still, there will be times when you want to act alone, when you want to test your own limits and see just how much you can accomplish. When you do, tell your lupus buddy or other trusted friend or family member what you intend to do so that he or she can lend help if need be. For example, if you are absolutely set on traveling by yourself, make sure that someone has your full itinerary and a way to reach you, just to check in.

Of course, other people cannot do everything for you. They cannot instill in you the determination to get past a difficult time, and they cannot force you to have a positive outlook in the midst of pain and suffering. But others can, by their presence in your life, help you understand that you are cared for, and that knowledge can, in turn, give you an anchor of hope on which to rely.

Support is most useful when it is given freely and received graciously. Keep this in mind as you go through the ups and downs of lupus flares and complications. Don't be afraid to ask, and don't be afraid to receive. And then, when you are feeling up to it, give whatever you can to someone else who is in need.

Where to Turn for Information

Whether you were diagnosed yesterday or five years ago, you will constantly be on the lookout for information about your disease, coping skills, and the latest in medical and medicinal discoveries. Filtering through all the information you find will take patience, objectivity, and reliance upon your and your doctor's sense of what is true and right for you.

Medical Breakthroughs

It seems as though each day there is a news story about a brilliant new breakthrough in the treatment of one or another disease. So-called cures are cropping up all the time, and alternative-medicine treatments are touted as "infallible" for the treatment of a myriad of ailments, including lupus.

How can you sift through all these exciting news items about the "latest medical miracle" to find things that will work for you in a safe, productive, and lasting way?

Many lupus organizations sponsor Web sites that post the latest in lupus research. These sites also post information about new medicines, treatments, and approaches to coping with symptoms. As you consult these sites, keep in mind that all information, especially news regarding new medications and treatments, should be reviewed by your doctor before you make use of it. Remember that each lupus patient is different; what is right for one person might not be right for another. Also, beware of anyone who assures you that he or she has *the* cure. When there is a true cure, you'll hear it from all the lupus organizations, your doctor, and other reputable sources first.

Ongoing Information

Several publications keep the lupus patient informed about the latest in medical breakthroughs, as well as treatments, tips for easier living, and personal growth. These include "Arthritis Today," a monthly publication of the Arthritis Foundation, "Lupus News," a quarterly publication of the Lupus Foundation of America, and several regional and local Lupus Foundation chapters' newsletters. In addition, there are newsletters published by "sister disease" organizations that offer informative articles, too. One such organization is the Sjögren's Syndrome Foundation, which publishes the newsletter "The Moisture Seekers," and the Scleroderma Foundation, which also publishes a newsletter, "Scleroderma Voice."

The LFA and the Arthritis Foundation have excellent pamphlets on topics ranging from "Laboratory Tests Used in the Diagnosis of Lupus" and "Joint and Muscle Pain in Systemic Lupus Erythematosus" (both published by LFA) to "Lupus: A Guide to Diagnosis and Treatment" (published by the Arthritis Foundation). Also, the National Institutes of Health publish information periodically, including their "Handbook on Health: Systemic Lupus Erythematosus," issued by NIH, National Institute of Arthritis and Musculoskeletal and Skin Diseases (NIAMS). You may receive these publications from the organizations themselves. Some are free and some are available for a nominal fee.

Books are another good source of information, but you must make sure that the edition you consult is current. *Dubois' Systemic Lupus Erythematosus*, 5th Edition (Baltimore, MD: Williams & Wilkins, 1997), edited by Daniel Wallace, M.D., and Bevra Hahn, M.D., is a comprehensive textbook on lupus and, although it is highly technical, can give you all the details of a particular aspect of the disease. Dr. Wallace is also the author of *The Lupus Book*, (Oxford University Press, 2000), which is an excellent medical guide for patients and their families.

To get the most thorough information, you should select a book that has been published recently (within the last three years). Look for books that have been endorsed by reputable organizations, such as the American College of Rheumatology, the LFA, or the Arthritis Foundation, so that you can have better assurance of getting accurate information from them.

If you are like most lupus patients, you do not have the funds to assemble an entire medical library. By joining a few lupus buddies, or your whole support group, you can start a lending library of texts that will be helpful to everyone. Also, the organizations that publish the pamphlets usually offer books for a reduced price, or make them available through their own lending library.

Where to Turn for More Help

If you need an adapted version of a specific appliance, gadget, or accommodation, contact the manufacturer of whatever it is you need and ask if they might develop something for you. Many companies, especially those that manufacture items made for a certain population, will be happy to listen to your suggestions, and you might come up with something that will benefit lupus sufferers the world over!

Also, adapting gadgets and other items that you already have can be a creative and inexpensive way to fashion something that is just right for you. One lupus patient lifts steaming pots and pans with her arms because her hands aren't strong enough—and she uses barbecue mitts that cover her hands, wrists, and elbows to accomplish it!

Each year, one lupus support group has an evening devoted to gadgets and gizmos. The members bring in tools, clothing, and suggestions for things that have helped them. The evening is a huge success, with each member taking away one or more new ideas to make his or her life that much easier.

Benefits and Pitfalls of Belonging to a Lupus Support Group

Organizations formed to assist patients with lupus include grass-roots support groups composed of a facilitator and members who have all been diagnosed with lupus of varying severity and with a myriad of different symptoms. These groups help the individual patient to feel that he or she is not alone in the fight against this mysterious illness with often no externally visible signs.

On the other hand, lupus is an extremely heterogeneous disease with disease manifestations and prognoses that vary from person to person over time. It may thus be unsettling to find that other people with similar symptoms and signs have been told that their outcome is better than yours. You will also see patients with varying degrees of disability due to different disease manifestations and due to varying ability to cope with symptoms. You cannot generalize about these situations, and you must rely on your doctor's assessment of your illness and your skills with dealing with adversity and illness.

National and state support organizations deal with fund-raising, research, and promoting lupus awareness in the community. In my opinion, I feel that sponsors of other rheumatic illnesses such as rheumatoid arthritis and osteoporosis have done a much better job of creating awareness of their illnesses and increasing funding of tax dollars for research. A more cohesive effort among individual lupus chapters in raising consciousness of lupus, its symptoms, and their chronicity will bring about earlier diagnoses and a concerted search for a cure for this unpredictable and highly variable illness.

You Are Impressive, Too!

As one of the men or women members of the lupus community, you are also unique, resilient, and creative when it comes to dealing with your disease and environment. In the moments when you are most in pain, troubled, or challenged by your disease, remember this fact and glean strength and inspiration from it—you are impressive, too!

18

THE FAITH FACTOR:

The Role of Spirit in Coping with Change

One of your greatest sources of support and protection against the vagaries of change due to lupus is your connection with your spirituality. If you can get to and achieve a sense of acceptance, peace, and even joy, you will be able to withstand all that lupus throws at you. Even more important, nurturing a spiritual life can help you cope with the challenges and changes of lupus. Lupus may wreak havoc with your body and way of life, but it has no power over your spirit or peace of mind. Spiritual practice makes it possible for you to take charge of your peace of mind despite lupus.

Faith Factor

With all the emotional upheavals that the diagnosis brings, and all the subsequent traumas that come from living with a chronic disease, having an inner core, a place of solace and retreat, is vital to your well-being. Moreover, some clinical studies have shown that patients with a sense of the spiritual have a greater chance of getting over illness more quickly and lengthening the periods of remission between bouts or flares. Through reading, developing relationships with others who strive for depth of spirit, and the support of a faith-centered community, you can get ever closer to your inner peace. You will also be able to draw upon the strength you find within when your lupus flares or other troubles in life surface.

Engaging a Belief System

If you already participate in an organized religion or other spiritual endeavors and include prayer, meditation, or quiet reflection in your daily activities, be vigilant in maintaining your connection with it. Connecting with the inner self, the spirit that is untouched by lupus, can be amazingly healing in its reminder of who you truly are.

Rabbi Levi Meier says, "Medical illness, emotional illness, and awareness of one's mortality determine greatly who you are. How you cope with those things is very important."

Rabbi Meier cautions, however, that spirituality is not about trying to find a cure for our illness in faith. "There is a difference," he says, "a distinction between 'curing' and 'healing.' The word 'heal' in its etymology means 'to become more whole.' So if you are ill, it is very possible to heal yourself, to become more whole, through spiritual pursuits, even if you are not cured.

"This entails a lot of time alone, in prayer both spontaneous and structured, in the analysis of dreams, and in spiritual analysis with a spiritual leader." The spiritual leader can be one individual or a group. A spiritual connection with others can bring you great emotional and physical support within it. Also, Rabbi Meier believes that reading good literature can promote spiritual growth and health.

A church or synagogue community can provide you with supportive fellowship, too, through communal prayer and assistance in managing your daily challenges. Attending services can provide you with a non-health-related outlet, and spiritual ritual and song can lift up your tired spirits and take you out of your suffering, if only for the moment.

Beyond these prayers, too, there is a world of spirituality that delves within as well as beyond articulated vocabulary. Through reading, developing relationships with others who strive for depth of spirit, and support of a faith-centered community, you can get ever closer to your inner peace. You will also be able to draw upon the strength you find within when your lupus flares or other troubles in life surface.

Seeking out Spiritual Practice

If you do not have a specific religious belief, begin to reach out and learn more about different spiritual practices and systems. This can be a wonderful and exciting part of your lupus journey. Explore spirituality as a way to get in touch with the strength and health that is all around you. Find a power greater than yourself with which to forge a relationship of trust and faith. For example, reconnect with nature, or develop a renewed appreciation for the world around you. Realize that the battle that is being waged within you can be made less strenuous when you are in partnership with spirit. Many spiritual traditions recognize the divine as love, and there is no greater force for healing than that.

Internalize your search for spiritual practice, too. Spend time in a comfortable, calming place, and open your heart to the options available to you, silently asking for guidance and dedication to your quest. Listen carefully and diligently for the answers to your searching questions.

When you attend religious services, gauge your inner reaction to them. Do you get the most out of rituals that are boisterous and praiseful, or quiet and contemplative? Do you feel more nurtured in a crowd of worshipers, or do you prefer a smaller gathering? Most important: Do you feel welcomed and cared about, do you feel loved, lupus and all?

Prayer

"There have been several studies regarding the connection between prayer and healing," says Father Frank Desiderio, C.S.P., a Roman Catholic priest and producer of the documentary *Healing and Prayer* for the Arts and Entertainment Network. "One such study showed that people with a religious practice tended to heal faster than those who did not."

There is a physiological reason for this phenomenon.

"Prayer invokes a relaxation response," says Desiderio. "And when you relax, you relieve stress."

Prayer, or its close kin, meditation, need not be formal and it need not be frequent.

"There are two components to praying," says Desiderio. "First, you establish a repetitive word or phrase that focuses your intro-spection. You use it to bring you back to your focus when your mind wanders. Second, you repeat the word or phrase, or do the activity, while breathing deeply."

Deep breathing, too, gives one the sense of cleansing and re-laxing.

"The most effective prayer is 'Thy will be done,' " says Deside-rio. "You can't control God; you can't force him to heal you. But you can pray for acceptance and peace."

In fact, making a laundry list of wants and offering them to God works against developing a close, trusting relationship with him. How, for example, are you going to feel if none of your petitions is answered the way you want? Also, if your way to pray consists only of asking God for things, in some ways, how will you benefit from the quietness of contemplation and, as a result, how will you be able to achieve true, strong inner peace?

Structured prayer (memorized or read prayers, repeated phrases, chanting, etc.) is one way to get away from a straight "wish list" to something deeper. Most of the world's religions, including Chris-tianity, Judaism, and Buddhism, have a strong tradition of struc-tured prayer that includes psalms of praise, deep emotion, and petition.

Prayers from a Lupus Patient's Perspective

Prayer is the most important element in my being able to cope with lupus. During the day, in the midst of all the struggles I face, I frequently lift up the prayer "Thy will be done." Also, I pray in other ways, depending on what I perceive to be my spiritual and physical needs. Here are some prayers that I have found helpful in my life with lupus. I begin each one by saying, "Dear Father in heaven," or "Dear Lord."

Praiseful Prayer

Today I am grateful for so many things.
I can move. I can talk. I can breathe.
I can sense the beautiful, wondrous world around me,
And for all these things, I am happy,
Deeply, genuinely happy,
In spite of lupus.
I wish to make the most of today.
Please help me to continue to appreciate this day,
To minister to my health in all ways,
And to feel this joy in all things great and small.

Prayer for a Loved One

I know that I am not the only person facing challenges.
In this moment, I lift up [NAME OF LOVED ONE]
With all the love and gratitude in my heart.
I pray that I will find ways to be as constant
And great a friend as he/she is to me.

Prayer for Taking a Step toward a Goal

Today, I moved closer to [GOAL].
It feels wonderful to be on my way,
And I am thankful for the energy, perseverance, and courage
It took me to get this far.
I am eager to take the next step
In health and happiness.

Prayer When You're in Pain

I am in terrible pain.
Today I ask for patience to endure my suffering.
Let me not be consumed by it,
But rather more courageous to face it and bear it out.
And let me rely on my loved ones and you, Lord,
To help me make it through.

Prayer When You're Afraid of the Future

I can't see the days before me.
I fear I have lost my way in darkness.
Give me calmness, a peaceful heart, and more faith
In my course of treatment, the wisdom of others,
And the inner strength you give me.
Together, I know that the darkness can become light!

Prayer for Health-care Professionals
Please give my doctors wisdom, good health,
Patience, and humor.
Endow them with the ability to discern what my symptoms mean
And how to treat them.
Steady the hands and eyes of those who run lab tests.
Grace all researchers with creativity and foresight.

Prayer of Saint Francis
(Prayer for Being of Use to Others)
Lord, make me an instrument of your peace.
Where there is hatred, let me sow love;
Where there is injury, pardon;
Where there is discord, unity;
Where there is doubt, faith;
Where there is despair, hope;
Where there is darkness, light;
Where there is sadness, joy.
O Divine Master,
Grant that I may not so much seek to be consoled
As to console;
To be understood
As to understand;
To be loved
As to love.
For it is in giving that we receive;
It is in pardoning that we are pardoned;
It is in dying that we are born to eternal life.
Amen

Reaching Out

A lupus support group or other nurturing, regular gathering can provide you with spiritual sustenance, too. Choose a group that is easily accessible to you (driving a long distance to and from could bring more aggravation than peace), and one that is well organized without being too controlled. Make sure that each person who wants to is given the chance to share without being dismissed. Gauge how you feel at the end of the meeting; you should be happier rather than more worried. Be sure you feel comfortable bringing your concerns to the group and are satisfied with the feedback and support you receive.

Positive Living

Another very important aspect of nurturing your spiritual side is to recognize those things that encourage you to deviate from your peaceful center.

It is easy to become despondent, or even depressed, by all the negative news and information available to us on a daily basis. Ask yourself if it is necessary to listen to all the terrible news on the television or radio. Tell people around you that you would rather talk about pleasant topics, and turn the conversation away from depressing subjects yourself if they seem unwilling or unable to.

Engage in activities that are good for you in a wholesome, healing sense, and, again, try to reduce the stress of negative or anger-sparking influences.

This does not mean that you ignore the realities of the world around you; nor does it mean that you sever ties with everyone in your life who does not take a positive approach to their relationship with you. But it does mean that you look upon your environment as medicine, another treatment to help you combat the war that is raging within you. The more you expose yourself to positive influences, the more you will absorb them and enable them to work upon you in a healing manner.

Practical ways that you can reduce some stress and negativity from your life include:

- Running errands at off hours when the stores and roads are less crowded
- Reading the newspaper instead of watching the televised news, which includes graphic visuals along with the stories
- Spreading out shopping for holiday and birthday gifts so that you are not stressed at what are supposed to be festive times
- Keeping encouraging pictures and sayings visible in your home and workplace
- Reading humorous or uplifting books
- Listening to soothing, pleasant music

- Watching children play
- Walking your dog
- Admiring the world around you, especially the beauty of nature
- Hiring others to do chores or errands for you when you feel overwhelmed, in a flare, or even when you feel fine

The Ups and Downs of Lupus— Tomorrow Is Another Day

Realizing that flares come and go, and that you will have times of relative calm and upset, will help you cope with the times when you are in pain and fighting your symptoms.

One lupus patient, who has had central nervous system (CNS) involvement, a heart attack, and kidney disease, says, "Things have been bad. Real bad. But I know that no matter how bad they are, there is a light at the end, a rainbow after the storm."

The Importance of Support Groups and Spiritual Nurturing in Lupus

The only thing worse than dealing with an unpredictable illness such as lupus is to have to cope with the unusual symptoms alone. Even the most supportive spouse or friend may fail to fathom how a lupus patient really feels. A support group helps one to hear stories of other affected peers, provides reassurance that one is not alone in his or her fight against lupus, and reduces the sense of isolation.

The best drugs and treatment for lupus do not offer perfect healing of the manifestations of lupus, and one needs to transfer the burden of residual fatigue or pain to a higher source in order to move on toward one's goals in life. The clergy and Eastern philosophies and practices of meditation and exercises can help you achieve inner peace and harmony and release powerful inner-healing forces.

In line with many studies that have shown the effect that remote prayer has on patient survival, it is only a matter of time before health practitioners may be mandated to offer a prayer along with traditional methods of treatment in order to ensure every possible chance of curing a patient's ailment.

19

Facing the Future

What is in store for lupus patients five, ten, twenty years from now? Will there be new medications that do not have awful side effects? Will there be greater public awareness so that lupus patients aren't constantly frustrated by insensitive comments and reactions?

Will there be a cure?

Healthy Developments

Although there is no cure for lupus today, there is hope. There are more research studies being funded and performed, as well as more understanding about the root causes of lupus, than ever before.

What Does a Study Do?

A study can revolve around the causes for lupus, treatments for certain symptoms, or new ways to combat the disease's progression and sometimes debilitating course. Studies can be aimed at quantitative analyses of data already available, or they can be developed around certain new parameters with either animal or human subjects. For example, a study might try to determine if a particular medication is effective against one or more lupus symptoms, or it might be focused on finding the correct dosage of the medication once its efficacy has been determined.

How Many Studies Are There?

Unfortunately, the number of lupus studies is small compared with the number of people who suffer from the disease. This is because of the lack of public awareness of lupus and the overwhelming awareness of other ailments. Until recently, there was not a concerted effort to centralize data indicating the number of people diagnosed with lupus. Even now, with more concrete numbers indicating a growing trend in diagnoses, lupus is still considered an "orphan disease," meaning the number of people perceived to suffer from it is not great enough to warrant extensive research and development.

Of course, other diseases such as cancer, AIDS, and multiple sclerosis need to be researched and funded, too. However, given the actual and growing number of people affected by lupus, it is reasonable to expect that more funding and studies should be available to find treatments for current symptoms and, eventually, a cure.

Will I Ever Be Part of a Study?

Publications such as the Lupus Foundation's newsletter and the Arthritis Foundation's magazine, *Arthritis Today*, as well as their Web sites, list studies currently being performed and those looking for people to participate. Also, your doctor might know of studies going on in your area, or your local hospital might be conducting research in conjunction with a nearby medical school.

Usually, when a study requests participants, there are specific parameters required of the applicants. For example, participants might be required to come from one geographic area, suffer from a specific symptom in lupus—say, kidney disease or pericarditis (inflammation of the lining of the heart)—or have other family members who also have autoimmune disease. In all cases, however, participation in studies is voluntary.

What Does a Study Entail?

Sometimes, after someone has been accepted into a study, participation consists of filling out a questionnaire regarding his or her family history of autoimmune disease, symptoms, medications, reactions to those medications, etc. Other times, a person is asked to take part in a clinical trial of new medication or other treatments (for example, natural remedies). In this case, researchers might be trying to find out what dosage of a particular medication will be effective, or what combination of substances will make up the medication that will, eventually, be developed.

Who Pays for Studies?

When you participate in a study, you are rarely charged; however, you might incur some cost if the medication or other substance being tested is not covered by conventional insurance. Sometimes participants are compensated for their time and effort. The compensation is not substantial, but it usually covers the participant's time and transportation cost.

Studies are funded by a variety of sources, usually a combination of more than one. These sources include learning institutions (universities, teaching hospitals) and government grants, pharmaceutical companies, and private donations, both large and small. Indeed, even the smallest donation can make a difference when added to the funds already available for research.

Overlapping Assistance

Because lupus shares so many symptoms and treatments with other illnesses, those who suffer from it can benefit from research carried out to better understand lupus's "cousins." For example, the great strides made recently to develop better nonsteroidal anti-inflammatory drugs (NSAIDs) used in treating osteoarthritis and rheumatoid arthritis have yielded better NSAIDs for lupus patients, too. Along the same lines, medications used to treat gastroesophageal reflux disease (GERD) and other gastrointestinal complaints have made a huge difference for lupus patients; in many cases, use of these medications has prevented patients from developing ulcers due to the mixture of other meds needed to control the lupus.

Diagnostic tools, used to define and quantify a variety of conditions, are becoming more precise for lupus symptoms and developments. As a result, physicians can pinpoint the area of concern much more easily than ever before. Blood tests especially are more sophisticated. Besides tracking antinuclear antibodies (ANA), tests can now reveal changes in neurological antibodies that could signal central nervous system involvement. They can also help refine a diagnosis of lupus to a more specific one of, for example, mixed connective tissue disease or Sjögren's syndrome.

Ultra–high resolution CAT scans are used more frequently to discern changes in lung tissue, as well as arterial complications, in some cases enabling intervention before severe lung or heart involvement occurs. Ultrasounds can show liver problems, as well as other organ abnormalities, without having to subject the patient to more invasive procedures.

New Developments in Treating Systemic Lupus Erythematosus

Great strides have been made in the last fifty years in the understanding of the normal functioning of the immune system and the problems that ensue when immune regulatory systems go awry. Proteins on the surface of the immune cells that help cells communicate with each other have been identified and cloned, and specific antibodies to these precise proteins have been synthesized and are in trials. Systemic lupus is at the crossroads at which rheumatoid arthritis was ten years ago. Just as the early treatments in rheumatoid arthritis showed some promise but were too toxic, some of the recent "smart drugs" for lupus have shown unusual side effects or have had to be tailored to specific lupus subsets. But etanercept and infliximab are two success stories for rheumatoid arthritis that resulted from the trials of numerous drugs against biological targets in cells.

Other novel treatments in development and trials are columns that can cleanse the blood of harmful antibodies and proteins that help to delete harmful clones of cells in lupus patients. Advances in transplantation and immunotherapy for cancer are yielding new treatments in organ-threatening lupus.

New Medications and Treatments

Some people are wary of trying new medications and treatments, even after they have been evaluated by organizations such as the Food and Drug Administration (FDA). It is true that many drug interactions and other side effects might not be readily known about some new medicines, but you can have a high degree of confidence that once a drug has been approved, the chances of suffering terrible effects from it are minimal.

New Drugs and What They Mean to You

In the United States, new medications undergo a rigorous cycle of research studies and scrutiny by private and governmental agencies. Because so much money and time are invested in bringing a new drug to market, pharmaceutical companies are prudent to make sure that a drug is safe. The FDA is also concerned about side effects. Although sometimes it "fast-tracks" a drug so that the people who need it can benefit from it more quickly, it, too, conducts rigorous tests and reviews of findings before it allows a drug to be marketed in the United States. It will also take a drug off the market if there are significant side effects that can be associated with it.

If your doctor prescribes a new drug, be sure you ask him or her what the potential side effects might be. Talk to your pharmacist, who is often able to give you an idea of the scope or frequency of side effects among the people to whom he or she dispenses the drug. Keep close track of any new symptoms you develop after starting the drug and report them to your doctor immediately. Be firm if you cannot tolerate a drug at all; the idea is to feel better, not worse! And pay close attention to the news and speak with your doctor if any stories arise that raise questions about the safety of a new drug.

Drugs in Other Countries

Each nation has its own policy toward medications. In some cases, most medications are available without a prescription. In others, a doctor must prescribe them. Some drugs that are not available in the United States can be legally obtained abroad for use by patients here. Consult with your doctor about treatments not readily available in the United States.

Under no circumstances should you take anything without discussing it first with your doctor. There could be side effects not reported in the country where you got the drug, or there could be unforeseen drug interactions with what you are already taking.

The World around You

Never before have there been so many helpful tools, accommodations, and new products for people suffering from disabilities. From clothes to carry-ons, life is definitely easier than it was even ten years ago—and it will keep getting better.

One of the reasons for this is the aging of the American population. By 2002, 50 percent of the people living in the United States will be age fifty or older. With this "graying of America" will come a larger group of individuals who need help with their daily lives. These people will exert more pressure on manufacturing, service, and governmental organizations to adapt their products and other offerings to their specific needs. Lupus patients will be a part of this groundswell of consumer demand, and will benefit from it, too. As America ages, lupus patients will find more products and services geared toward making their lives easier.

Another reason for the increasingly improved quality of life comes from the attitude of so many disabled people—the attitude of not giving up and not giving in. This goes beyond the current laws and ordinances demanding more accommodation in public places and the workplace, and it goes beyond the "healthy" population reaching out to help those less fortunate. Rather, it goes right to the core of each individual's personal strength and faith. If someone believes that he or she can do something, there will be a way to do it, and the knowledge gained by one person's experience can educate and inspire a whole new generation of active, determined people.

It used to be that someone who suffered from a chronic illness or was physically disabled couldn't do very much except stay at home. Now, people with disabilities travel all over the world, compete in athletic events, write poetry, run businesses, and contribute productively and significantly to the world around them. Not everyone with a disability can work, and that will probably always be the case. But the perception of the disabled person as helpless is very outdated and has been replaced by a dynamic, ever-achieving community of people who, no matter what their ailments or weaknesses, can find strength and meaning in the world around them.

Creating More Awareness for Systemic Lupus Erythematosus

Symptoms and signs of systemic lupus may be subtle and not always visible or measurable, such as they are in rheumatoid arthritis or osteoporosis. Better studies aimed at measuring severity and quality of life in lupus and creating disease-specific measurements for various symptoms and signs will help to demonstrate the significant impact of this illness on people's lives.

It takes an average of three years after the onset of lupus symptoms in an adult to establish a diagnosis. The reason is multifactorial and includes the facts that the symptoms are not specific, that awareness of lupus is limited except among specialists, and that tests often have to be considered in light of how noteworthy the symptoms are. Joint pains in the small fingers of the hands and/or rashes on the face, upper extremities, and torso are the first symptoms in up to 70 percent of lupus patients, usually women. A useful acronym and phrase to describe this would be: "Little joints hurting or Unusual Peeling Ulcers or Skin rash constitute a 'lupus attack' unless proven otherwise." If such acronyms can be spread effectively among primary-care physicians, then lupus can be diagnosed earlier and more effective treatment instituted to prevent complications such as kidney, heart, or brain involvement.

Your Personal Future

As you read about all the strides that science, medicine, and others with chronic illnesses have made, you will probably wonder what all this means to you. The answer to this question resides in your own heart and soul: You will be able to make of your future what you choose to make of it.

Realistically, this means that you probably won't be able to cure yourself of lupus. However, it does mean that the attitudes you have toward your illness and other aspects of your life, the people you surround yourself with, the things you do and think each day and night are completely within your control. And with this control comes the key to what your personal future will be like.

Death and Lupus

When you were diagnosed, you probably asked your doctor what the chances were of your dying from lupus. This is a natural response to finding out that you have a disease for which there is no cure, and which might progress into severely debilitating symptoms.

The answer to that question is reassuring: People with mild lupus (non-organ-threatening lupus) can usually look forward to a normal life span. For those patients with organ-threatening disease, the odds are ever better that they, too, will live a long time after diagnosis, thanks to new medications and treatments and earlier intervention.

Still, you will hear stories of someone who had lupus and died. These stories are not to be taken lightly; however, they need not color how you look at your future. Each lupus patient is different, just as are the circumstances surrounding his or her medical care, disease progression, and attitude toward care. You need to do all that you can to give yourself a healthful, meaningful life so that you can maximize your chances of living to your fullest enjoyment possible. You need to keep your attitude fixed on the future, and not dwell too much on the possibility of dying from lupus.

Everyone will die someday, whether or not lupus is a factor. Accept this inevitable aspect of being human. Face your fears and thoughts about death, and reconcile your spiritual side to this fact of human mortality.

Then forge ahead into the future.

What about You?

Ask yourself about the kind of future you want to have inside, the kind of spirit you want to live with day in and day out. Is it one of resilience? Hope? Determination? Triumph? Start now by cultivating the aspects of your life that bring you joy, peace, and an abiding faith.

Do you want to reach out to the world and do all you can to maintain your friends and support system, and nurture your family? Then learn to be a friend and a supportive member of your family and faith community in spite of lupus. Learn your limits and the extent to which you can reach out and give to others. Learn when to say no and when to say yes.

Do you have educational, professional, or leisure goals? Examine them carefully, take stock of your health and emotional resources, and then make a plan to achieve them, even with lupus. It might take you more time than you'd originally thought, or you might have to modify your goals to accommodate your present reality. There will be times when life, and lupus, will "intervene." But there is no reason why you should shelve your dreams forever.

Life with Lupus Is a Journey

Finally, in this age of instantly getting from point A to point B, whether through flight or Internet connections, we have lost a bit of the wonder and adventure of the journey.

Life with lupus is a journey. It is full of surprises, twists and turns, pain and achievement. Along the way, you will meet incredibly gifted people and learn to know yourself intimately, inside and out. You will suffer setbacks, hardships, and losses. You will become lost in denial for a time. And you will be frustrated and angry sometimes, too.

But you will also acquire amazing strength, deep grace, and an appreciation for life, simple life, that is unparalleled. You will develop some of the strongest relationships you have ever known, and you will be witness to many triumphs in your life and those of your loved ones. You will also discover a world of spirituality that is personal, deep, and true, and you will be given opportunities to help others and give them a sense of hope and strength through your example and care.

As you grow and change, your journey will take on new meaning to you and those around you. You won't always understand the implications of what happens to you or others, but you will never doubt the impact of your life upon others and how your attitude impresses and inspires.

Whether you were diagnosed yesterday or three years ago, you will see that your lupus journey will be a unique reflection of yourself and all the things you are and can be. A gift, as well as a life and a journey.

Are you ready for it?

Yes, you are.

Now, begin.

SPECIAL ADDITION

Frequently Asked Questions and Answers

In writing this book, we encountered many men and women who were generous with their time and stories about coping with lupus. In addition to their comments, they had many questions about the disease and certain aspects of their lives with lupus. In thanks to them for their time and candor, we have included their questions here. We hope they will find the answers helpful to meeting and overcoming their daily challenges.

1. *I'm feeling better, so why can't I just stop taking my medicine?*
   Some medications can act so subtly that you don't notice their effects until you stop taking them. Others protect you from the effects of symptoms that would otherwise be out of control. Before stopping any medication, or changing your dosage, you should always consult your doctor. Also, you should always report any side effects to your doctor immediately, even if you think the effects are minor. Beyond these important points, you need to remember that lupus is a chronic illness, so you will always have to monitor it and take appropriate steps prescribed and supervised by your doctor to ensure that your symptoms are kept under control as much as possible.

2. *If my lab results look so good, why do I still feel awful?*
   Lab results usually measure whether one has an abnormal blood count or abnormal liver, kidney, and electrolyte levels.

Further blood tests, such as a sedimentation rate (ESR), complement levels, and antibody levels such as double-stranded DNA antibody, vary during increases in disease activity and may rise or fall. However, in non-organ-threatening lupus, many of these tests are only moderately abnormal and often remain within normal limits. In these situations, disturbances of the autonomic nervous system—which regulates blood flow to every organ in the body and controls the activity of the heart, intestines, and lungs—cause the innumerable symptoms of muscle and joint pain, dizziness, nausea, alternating diarrhea and constipation, and shortness of breath. This is not usually from active lupus and needs to be treated with specific medications and therapies.

3. *Why do prescription medications cost so much?*
Publicly held drug companies are answerable to their shareholders to turn a profit. They also must invest a great deal of time, money, and resources into developing medications and marketing them to be sure people are aware of their availability and benefits. These factors contribute significantly to the cost of the medications that are available to patients. Although the cost of prescription drugs can be very high, in many cases the benefits they bring outweigh the monetary sacrifice.

4. *Some people attribute all their ailments to lupus. Is this reasonable?*
Lupus is a multisystem illness, and, as mentioned in the earlier question, disturbances in the autonomic nervous system can bring out widespread symptoms. However, the diagnosis of any illness brings on some degree of increased vigilance over one's body, and hence it is very reasonable that one may attribute some normal musculoskeletal twinges to lupus. Some estimates have shown that the average healthy person experiences some musculoskeletal pain every fourth day of his or her normal life.

5. *Why isn't there a cure yet?*
Lupus is one of the most complex, difficult-to-understand diseases known to man. Before there is a cure, all the components of the disease (genetic components, triggers, symptoms, progression) must be classified, understood, and put in the context of currently available medical treatments and protocols. It's a very intricate problem, but one that is going to be unraveled someday!

6. *If I have lupus, will I be more likely to get cancer?*

Incidences of cancer in lupus patients are the same as in the general population. Some immunosuppressive drugs can increase a lupus patient's propensity to develop certain cancers, but, again, the numbers of these cases are small.

7. *Can lupus patients take any prescription or over-the-counter medicine or herbal medication?*

Lupus patients must first check with their doctors before taking any prescription or over-the-counter medicine or herbal medication. Checking with a reputable pharmacist is also a good idea. Even so-called natural preparations can interact with each other and exacerbate certain symptoms (such as depression). Also, some decongestants and antihistamines can have harmful side effects when mixed with other prescription drugs, alcohol, or over-the-counter medicines. Some herbal medications such as echinacea can stimulate an already overactive immune system and should be avoided.

8. *Are generic and brand-name prescription medications the same?*

Certain brand medications differ from their generic counterparts in the rate and extent of absorption due to differences in the coating or the fillers employed in making the generic medications. Examples of such medications include warfarin (Coumadin), used to treat blood-clotting disorders, L-thyroxine (Synthroid), used to treat an underactive thyroid, and diphenylhydantoin (Dilantin), used to treat seizures. In general, one can be treated with either the generic or brand-name medicine, provided one does not switch back and forth between the two. Anecdotal experience suggests that more rashes occur with generic hydroxychloroquine than its brand-name version (Plaquenil).

9. *My sister stays out in the sun all the time and never takes care of herself. I've always been careful about my health, and yet I'm the one who got lupus. Why?*

It is very important that you never blame yourself for getting lupus. Such an approach is counterproductive to maintaining a positive attitude while fighting your disease and symptoms. That said, it could be frustrating to see other people, who seemingly abuse their bodies, remain healthy while you suffer. Although scientists are still not sure what causes lupus, it is becoming clearer that there are genetic and environmental components that factor into developing the disease. Because each person is unique in terms of his or her environment and genetic makeup, even if you have a propensity for it, you might never develop lupus. Likewise, you could do everything right, and still develop the disease. Rather than feeling guilty or frustrated that you have lupus (or were unlucky enough to get it), dwell on the positives in your life and the need to do everything possible to maintain a productive outlook on who you are and what you can do in spite of lupus.

10. *I've heard that lupus disappears after menopause. Is that true?*

Changes in hormonal activity during menopause may take away the sharp decline in estrogen levels in the normal menstrual cycle, which is associated with low steroid production in the body. Low levels of internal steroid production may lead to less suppression of immune activity. Hence, theoretically lupus should improve after menopause, although this is not universally true.

11. *How do I know if I'm in remission?*

You can tell when you are in clinical remission when you have no symptoms or signs of activity of lupus, such as joint pain or protein in the urine, even though you may be on medication. Serological remission occurs when symptoms, signs of illness, and abnormal antibodies such as antinuclear antibodies also disappear. Your doctor is the best guide as to when it is safe for you to lower your medication dose.

12. *Do certain ethnic or racial groups have a greater chance of getting lupus?*

This is controversial, as some investigators have shown that a lower socioeconomic status and hence a decreased access to health care results in more severe and detectable lupus in African-American and Asian populations in the United States. Others have shown that the number of patients with lupus in these ethnicities is definitely higher than in Caucasians. This question will be answered better when all the genes and environmental factors contributing to the development of lupus are identified.

13. *Why do I feel terrible when the weather changes?*

The old adage is that the grandma's knee is a good meteorological instrument. Scientific studies have failed to validate this, but doctors see this too often for it to be coincidental. It is possible that adverse weather conditions may make it more difficult to cope with joint pain and hence increase the suffering.

14. *What jobs are best for lupus patients?*

The best jobs for lupus patients are those that will accommodate the steps they need to take to maintain a balance in their lives, as well as control over their treatments and symptoms. Jobs that are flexible are preferred, the kind of jobs where the patient is able to have control over his or her schedule and that provide a supportive, positive atmosphere. Above all, the lupus patient needs to enjoy the kind of work he or she does, and feel a sense of accomplishment and contribution as well.

15. *How can you be sure you have lupus? Whom do you believe when you get several opinions?*

Lupus can be a difficult disease to diagnose, particularly because all or some of the symptoms and signs might not occur at the same time. It is important to keep track of all your symptoms and make sure that your primary-care physician has them on record, too. Continue to pursue answers to your perplexing problems, and seek second opinions when you feel confused about the different "stories" you are getting about the reason for your symptoms. For a definitive diagnosis, rely on a qualified lupus specialist, almost always a rheumatologist, and be sure your diagnosis is based upon the criteria set forth by the American College of Rheumatology.

16. *Once you have an elevated ANA, should you repeat the test? Does it fluctuate? Do other test results (antibody tests) fluctuate?*

An antinuclear nuclear antibody (ANA) is of diagnostic importance because over 97 percent of patients with lupus will have a significantly positive test. Higher titers (that is, a high amount of ANA) correlate more with disease specificity rather than severity. In other words, the higher your ANA titer is, the more certain you can be that you have a significant autoimmune illness. Disappearance of an ANA suggests serological remission.

Other antibodies that fluctuate with disease activity include the double-stranded DNA antibody in kidney disease, and ribosomal P protein antibody in some cases of brain involvement. Often a sudden fall in titer indicates that a flare is imminent in the ensuing three months, as this indicates binding of antibodies to body tissues. The higher the titer of these antibodies, the more likely one is to have involvement of organs and systemic illness.

Complement proteins are made by the liver and play an important role in causing inflammation and tissue damage as directed by the immune system. A sudden fall in the levels suggests the possibility of a flare in the next three months.

17. *What role does diet play in lupus?*
There is no "lupus diet" designed to "cure" lupus. However, a well-balanced, nutritious diet is essential for maintaining good health. Avoid fad diets, or those that rely on one type of food exclusively. Report any marked weight loss or weight gain to your doctor immediately.

18. *How can I get Internet access if I don't have a computer at home?*
Most public libraries have computers that provide Internet access, and they make these available to their patrons. There are also Internet service providers that will give free mailbox service so you can send and receive e-mail, too.

19. *I have lupus and was just diagnosed with Sjögren's syndrome, too. How common is it to have more than one chronic illness? Can I expect to get anything else?*
A significant number of lupus patients will have features of a second autoimmune illness. For every six patients with lupus, one patient will have mixed connective tissue disease, which has features of lupus, muscle weakness from muscle inflammation, thickened hidebound skin in the hands suggestive of scleroderma, and high titers of a special antibody called ribonucleoprotein antibody. Similarly, among the 30 percent of lupus patients with the SSA antibody, more than half of them develop dry eye and mouth symptoms suggestive of Sjögren's syndrome. About 15 percent of lupus patients have issues with excessive blood clotting mediated by antibodies to phospholipid and protein compounds, which is called the antiphospholipid syndrome. Other lupus patients may have hypothyroidism, rheumatoid arthritis, or colitis.

20. *How do I know when I've "outgrown" my doctor and need to find someone else to treat my new/perplexing symptoms?*
If you are not getting any relief for your symptoms, or feel your doctor is not interested in continuing your care, you should at least seek a second opinion, if not change physicians. If your physician does not listen to your complaints, or ignores or misses indications of serious conditions in your symptoms or lab work, you should consider switching doctors. Also, if

your physician does not pursue continuing education in the field of rheumatology and, specifically, lupus, you should probably switch to a physician who will be better equipped to provide you with the latest treatments and news about your condition.

Glossary

Anti-inflammatory A medication given to reduce swelling and inflammation of tissues.

Arthralgia Pain in one or more joints.

Arthritis Inflammation of one or more joints.

Autoimmunity Allergy to one's own tissues.

Biopsy Removal of a bit of tissue for examination under a microscope. In lupus, kidney, lung, and/or skin biopsies are used to ascertain disease activity.

Brand-name drug The originating company's patented market name for a medication.

Chronic A persistent, ongoing condition.

Criteria Standards by which a judgment or diagnosis can be made.

Erythematosus Having a reddish hue.

Fatigue The feeling of being extremely, bone-wearily tired. Sometimes accompanied by muscle lethargy.

Fibromyalgia A pain-amplification syndrome usually characterized by fatigue, a sleep disorder, and specific tender "trigger points" located in the soft tissues.

Flare Exacerbation of disease activity; the reappearance of symptoms.

Generic drug A medication composed of the same active ingredients as the brand-name version, but which may be processed with different binding substances.

Hemagologic Of or pertaining to the blood.

Immunosuppressive   A substance or medication that treats lupus by suppressing, or slowing down, the immune system.

Malar rash   A reddish eruption usually across the cheeks and bridge of the nose that takes the shape of a flying butterfly. (Sometimes also called the "butterfly rash.")

Neurologic   Of or pertaining to the central nervous system.

NSAID   A nonsteroidal anti-inflammatory medication (an example is ibuprofin).

Photosensitivity   Reaction to ultraviolet light.

Prognosis   The prospect of survival and/or recovery from a disease.

Raynaud's phenomenon   A blue, white, or black discoloration of the hands or feet, especially in cold temperatures.

Renal   Of or pertaining to the kidneys.

Rheumatic disease   A disorder affecting the immune and/or musculoskeletal systems.

Thrombocytopenia   Low platelet count.

Toxic   Harmful and/or life threatening.

Serositis   Inflammation of one or more serious membranes, such as the pericardium (the sac around the heart) or the pleura (the sac around the lungs).

Sjögren's syndrome   A condition sometimes seen with lupus characterized by dry mouth, dry eyes, and arthritis. When Sjögren's syndrome appears by itself (without lupus), it is called primary Sjögren's.

Steroid   Anti-inflammatory hormones produced naturally by the adrenal cortex, or synthetically.

Sunscreen   A chemical substance that blocks out ultraviolet light.

Systemic   Of or pertaining to the body as a whole.

Trigger   An event or substance that can cause a disease to appear or a flare to erupt.

Helpful Resources

Organizations and Publications

The Lupus Foundation of America, Inc.
1300 Piccard Drive
Suite 200
Rockville, MD 20850-4303
Phone: 301-670-9292 • Fax: 301-670-9486
E-mail: LUPUSNEWS@aol.com • Web site: www.lupus.org
Newsletter: "Lupus News"

The Arthritis Foundation
P.O. Box 7669
Atlanta, GA 30357-0669
Phone: 1-800-207-8633 • Web site: www.arthritis.org
Arthritis Answers: 800-283-7800 • Magazine: *Arthritis Today*

Scleroderma Foundation
12 Kent Way
Suite 101
Byfield, Massachusetts 01922
Phone: 978-463-5843 • Fax: 978-463-5809
Info Line: 800-722-HOPE (4673)
E-mail: sfinfo@scleroderma.org
Web site: www.scleroderma.org • Newsletter: "Scleroderma Voice"

Sjögren's Syndrome Foundation, Inc.
366 North Broadway
Jericho, New York 11753
Phone: 516-933-6365 • Fax: 516-933-6368
Info Requests: 800-473-6473
Web site (with e-mail link): www.sjogrens.org
Newsletter: "The Moisture Seekers"

National Alopecia Areata Foundation
P.O. Box 150760
San Rafael, California 94915-0760
Phone: 415-456-4644 • Fax: 415-456-4274
E-mail: info@naaf.org • Web site: www.naaf.org

American College of Rheumatology
1800 Century Place
Suite 250
Atlanta, GA 30345
Phone: 404-633-3777 • Fax: 404-633-1870
E-mail: acr@rheumatology.org
Web site: www.rheumatology.org

**National Arthritis and Musculoskeletal and Skin Diseases
Information Clearinghouse**
**National Institute of Arthritis and Musculoskeletal and Skin
Diseases (NIAMS)**
National Institutes of Health
1 AMS Circle
Bethesda, MD 20892-3675
Phone: 301-496-8188 • Fax: 301-718-6366
TTY: 301-565-2966 • Web site: www.nih.gov/naims/
Publications: Various

American Medical Association
515 N. State Street
Chicago, Illinois 60610
Phone: 312-464-5000 • Web site: www.ama-assn.org
Publication: *The Journal of the American Medical Association*
Web site: www.jama.com

Products and Consumer Information

InfoGrip, Inc.
1794 E. Main Street
Ventura, CA 93001
Phone: 805-652-0770 • Toll-free: 800-397-0921
Fax: 805-652-0880 • E-mail: sales@infogrip.com
Web site: www.infogrip.com
Products: Computer peripherals and other office items designed
for persons with special needs.

Medic Alert Foundation
Phone: 888-633-4298 • Web site: www.medicalert.com

OXO International
1175 Ninth Avenue
5th Floor
New York, NY 10011
Phone: 212-242-3333 • Fax: 212-242-3336
Catalog orders by phone: 800-545-4411
E-mail: info@oxo.com • Web site: www.oxo.com
Products: Household tools and cooking gadgets designed for
people with arthritis and other special physical considerations.

Sun Precautions
2815 Wetmore Avenue
Everett, Washington 98201
Phone: 800-822-7860 • Fax: 425-303-0836
Web site: www.sunprecautions.com
Products: Sun-protective clothing, accessories, and sunscreen
products for adults and children.

Sun Solutions
P.O. Box 595
Woods Hole, Massachusetts 02543
Phone: 800-895-0010 • Fax: 508-540-1884
Web site: www.sunsolutionsclothing.com
Products: Sun-protective clothing for adults and children.

"tlc"
340 Poplar Street
Hanover, PA 17333-0080
Phone: 800-850-9445   •   Fax: 800-757-9997
Web site: www.tlccatalog.org
Products: Distributed by the American Cancer Society, this
catalog contains fashionable hats and other head coverings for
people experiencing hair loss.

Other Web Sites of Interest

www.assistance-dogs-intl.org
> Listing of organizations that train and place companion and
> assistance dogs.

www.cdc.gov
> Centers for Disease Control provides information on current
> health matters nationwide and travel areas where health issues
> are of particular concern.

www.disAbility.gov
> Web site set up by the United States government to give
> information on many aspects of the lives of the disabled.

www.medicare.gov
> Information concerning Medicare health benefits.

www.pcepd.gov
> President's Committee on Employment for People with
> Disabilities.

www.ssa.gov
> Web site of the United States Social Security Administration
> that provides information on applying for and working with
> Social Security benefits.

www.urbanlegends.about.com and www.snopes.com
> Source for the "real scoop" about health stories and other tales
> told via the Internet.

Suggested Reading

Larry Dossey, M.D., *Healing Words: The Power of Prayer and the Practice of Medicine.* HarperPaperbacks, 1993.

Harold G. Koenig, M.D., *The Healing Power of Faith.* Simon and Schuster, 1999.

Rabbi Levi Meier, *Ancient Secrets: Using the Stories of the Bible to Improve Our Everyday Lives.* Jewish Lights Publishing, 1996.

Daniel J. Wallace, M.D., and Bevra Hahn, M.D., editors, *Dubois' Systemic Lupus Erythematosus.* Williams & Wilkins, 1997.

Daniel J. Wallace, M.D., *The Lupus Book.* Oxford University Press, 2000.

Index

Abdominal pain, 6, 70
Acceptance, 42–43
Acupuncture, 63
Advocates, 74
Affirmations, positive, 16, 38
Age, lupus and, 6, 13
Alcohol consumption, 32, 47
Alopecia (see Hair loss)
Alpha hydroxy-butryic acid, 140
Alternative medicine, 63, 179,
    204
American College of Rheumatol-
    ogy (ACR), 6, 7, 54, 180,
    206
American Medical Association
    Web site, 54
Americans with Disabilities Act
    (ADA), 107
Anemia, 9, 138
Anger, 15, 22, 35, 165
    management of, 36–37
Antibiotic drugs, 78
Anti-inflammatory drugs, 79, 83
Antimalarial drugs, 50, 138
Antinausea drugs, 50
Antinuclear antibody (ANA), 9,
    195, 206
Anti-phospholipid syndrome,
    207
Anti-Rho antibody, 160

Anxiety, 34, 37
Appearance (see Personal factor)
Appetite loss, 50
Arthritis, 8, 133
Arthritis Foundation, 33, 34, 74,
    87, 90, 91, 98–99, 112, 134,
    136, 168, 176, 177, 179,
    180, 193
Aspirin, 79, 160
Assertiveness
    diplomatic, 58, 101–102
    lupus consumer and, 93
Autoimmune disease, lupus as, 5,
    6
Automobiles, 94–96
Azathioprine (Imuran), 50, 51

Ballroom dancing, 124
Bankruptcy, 91
Barter arrangements, 91
Bathrooms, 118–119
Bedrooms, 117–118
Big-ticket items, 94–99
Bladder disturbances, 34
Bleeding, 60
Blood sugar, 49
Blood tests, 49, 83, 195, 202–203
Body image, 15
Books, 180
Bowel disturbances, 34